THE BOOK BEHIND BILL CLINTON'S LIFE-CHANGING PLANT-BASED DIET

FEATURED IN THE NEW DOCUMENTARY FORKS OVER KNIVES

THE *NEW YORK TIMES* BESTSELLER

Wit 0
Gre s

Prevent *and* Reverse Heart Disease

The Revolutionary, Scientifically Proven, Nutrition-Based *Cure*

Caldwell B. Esselstyn, Jr., M.D.

Foreword by T. Colin Campbell, Ph.D., author of *The China Study*

"Proves that changes in diet (and that alone) cause radical changes in the age and disease of your arteries."

—Michael Roizen, M.D., coauthor of *You: On a Diet*

"Dr. Caldwell Esselstyn has directed pioneering research demonstrating that the progression of even severe coronary heart disease can often be reversed by making comprehensive changes in diet and lifestyle."

—Dean Ornish, M.D., founder, President, and Director, Preventive Medicine Research Institute, and author of *Dr. Dean Ornish's Program for Reversing Heart Disease*

"A hard-nosed scientist shows us his secrets for successfully cleaning the rusting arteries of so many patients—and it doesn't even hurt."

—Mehmet Oz, M.D., coauthor of *You: The Owner's Manual*

"Dr. Esselstyn has always been ahead of his time. His focus on the healing powers of proper nutrition on diseased coronary arteries has now proven right, raising another unthinkable notion—that heart patients can cure themselves."

—Bernadine Healy, M.D., former Director, National Institutes of Health

"This powerful program will make you virtually heart-attack-proof. On the basis of decades of research, Dr. Caldwell Esselstyn has shown not only how to prevent heart disease but also how to reverse it—even for people who have been affected for many years. I strongly recommend this important book."

—Neal D. Barnard, M.D., founder and President, Physicians Committee for Responsible Medicine, and author of *Breaking the Food Seduction*

"*Prevent and Reverse Heart Disease* provides a practical approach for people to regain their lost health. Considering the worldwide prevalence of coronary artery disease, this book should become the best-seller of all time."

—John A. McDougall, M.D., author of *The McDougall Program*

"Dr. Esselstyn's eminently successful arrest-and-reversal therapy for heart disease through patient education and empowerment as the treatment of choice will send shock waves through a mercenary medical system that focuses largely on pills and procedures."

—Hans Diehl, founder and Director, Coronary Health Improvement Project

"Dr. Esselstyn's solution in *Prevent and Reverse Heart Disease* is as profound as Newton's discovery of gravity. Half of all Americans dying today could have changed their date with the undertaker by following Dr. Esselstyn's plan."

—Howard F. Lyman, coauthor of *No More Bull!* and *Mad Cowboy*

"If you have heart disease, this book should be essential reading. It could save your life."

—Michael F. Jacobson, Executive Director, Center for Science in the Public Interest

Prevent and Reverse Heart Disease

THE REVOLUTIONARY, SCIENTIFICALLY PROVEN, NUTRITION-BASED *CURE*

CALDWELL B. ESSELSTYN, JR., M.D.

AVERY
A MEMBER OF PENGUIN GROUP (USA) INC.
New York

Published by the Penguin Group
Penguin Group (USA) Inc., 375 Hudson Street, New York, New York 10014, USA · Penguin Group (Canada), 90 Eglinton Avenue East, Suite 700, Toronto, Ontario M4P 2Y3, Canada (a division of Pearson Penguin Canada Inc.) · Penguin Books Ltd, 80 Strand, London WC2R 0RL, England · Penguin Ireland, 25 St Stephen's Green, Dublin 2, Ireland (a division of Penguin Books Ltd) · Penguin Group (Australia), 250 Camberwell Road, Camberwell, Victoria 3124, Australia (a division of Pearson Australia Group Pty Ltd) · Penguin Books India Pvt Ltd, 11 Community Centre, Panchsheel Park, New Delhi–110 017, India · Penguin Group (NZ), 67 Apollo Drive, Rosedale, North Shore 0632, New Zealand (a division of Pearson New Zealand Ltd) · Penguin Books (South Africa) (Pty) Ltd, 24 Sturdee Avenue, Rosebank, Johannesburg 2196, South Africa

Penguin Books Ltd, Registered Offices: 80 Strand, London WC2R 0RL, England

First trade paperback edition 2008

Illustration on page 41 and recipe illustrations by Ted Esselstyn
Figures 1, 13, 14 are reproduced, with permission, from C. B. Esselstyn, "Resolving the Coronary Artery Disease Epidemic Through Plant-Based Nutrition," *Preventive Cardiology*, 2001, 4:171–77; 2, 3, 16, 17 are reprinted with permission of the Cleveland Clinic Foundation; 15 is reproduced, with permission, from *Journal of Family Practice*, 1995, 41(6):560–68.

Published simultaneously in Canada

The Library of Congress catalogued the hardcover edition as follows:

Esselstyn, Caldwell B., date.
Prevent and reverse heart disease : the revolutionary, scientifically proven, nutrition-based cure / Caldwell B. Esselstyn, Jr.
p. cm.
Includes bibliographical references and index.
ISBN-13: 978-1-58333-272-6
ISBN-10: 1-58333-272-3
1. Coronary heart disease—Prevention. 2. Vegetarian cookery. 3. Nutrition. I. Title.
RC685.C6E77 2007 2006028947
616.1'2305—dc22

ISBN-13: 978-1-58333-300-6; ISBN-10: 1-58333-300-2 {paperback edition}

Printed in the United States of America
25 27 29 30 28 26 24

This book is dedicated to my wife, Ann Crile Esselstyn,
who gives everything meaning.

And to my original research patients,
who placed their faith in me.

Contents

Part Two. The Joy of Eating

Foreword

ONE MORNING IN THE SUMMER OF 1991, I received an interesting phone call from a surgeon at the prestigious Cleveland Clinic in Ohio. He had read a recent *New York Times* story about our study on diet, lifestyle, and health in China and was interested in our preliminary findings. He invited me to speak at a conference that fall in Tucson, Arizona. His ambitious title for the meeting: "The First National Conference on the Elimination of Coronary Artery Disease."

That, in itself, was intriguing enough to persuade me to accept. But I also was impressed by the fact that this Dr. Esselstyn had secured the participation of many well-known heart specialists, including Framingham Heart Study director William Castelli and Dr. Dean Ornish, who had recently gained considerable recognition for his work showing the possiblity of reversing heart disease through changes in diet and lifestyle. This conference would be challenging, to say the least. In my own academic environment, it was startling enough at the time even to mention a tenuous association of diet and heart disease. But the *elimination* of coronary artery disease? This was a paradigm shift.

The conference was highly successful—and provocative. So was a subsequent meeting in Orlando, Florida, which Dr. Esselstyn organized in association with Michael Eisner, then chief executive officer of the Walt Disney Company.

Since those early days, my wife, Karen, and I have come to know well both Dr. Esselstyn—"Essy," as his friends call him—and his energetic wife and colleague, Ann. I have often lectured with him on the same stage. And I have come to know his remarkable research and its findings, as well as its major implications.

Dr. Esselstyn's studies are among the most carefully conducted and relevant medical investigations undertaken during the past century. His goal—eliminating coronary disease entirely—may not be achievable during our lifetimes, but he has told us that it can be done and how it can be done. His determination to pursue this research and to teach the rest of us what he has learned, against formidable opposition in the medical establishment, is a testament to his personal and professional courage and integrity.

This book is a must read, both for ordinary people interested in health and for the dons of clinical and medical research institutions. People who ignore its message will do so at their own peril. There is no pharmaceutical wonder or medical trickery, either now or in the future, that can match these findings.

—T. Colin Campbell, professor emeritus of nutritional biochemistry, Cornell University, and coauthor of The China Study *(2005)*

Introduction

THIS BOOK HAS ITS ORIGINS in the dramatic experiences of twenty-three men and one woman who came to me in despair and without hope some twenty years ago. At the time, I was a surgeon at the renowned Cleveland Clinic. Year in and year out, the clinic is widely recognized as the number one heart center in the world. And indeed, there is no way to exaggerate the remarkable innovations and feats of surgical wonder that my colleagues have been able to introduce into the world of medicine.

But a surgeon has only so many tools to use against a lethal disease, and in the case of the patients to whom this book is dedicated, the clinic's physicians had found themselves in the position of having to say that there was nothing more they could do.

This is always the hardest moment both for the patient and the physician—the time when, in effect, a death sentence has been rendered. And that was the position the majority of these patients found themselves in back in 1985. They were, it must be acknowledged, a sorry lot by the time they arrived in my office—sorry in terms of both their physical health and their spirits.

Most demoralizing for those who had been the beneficiaries of the clinic's surgical interventions was the recognition that so much that had been done to save them—repeated open heart surgery, angioplasties aplenty, stents, and a host of medications—seemed no longer to have any useful effect. Almost all the men had lost their sexual potency. Most had chest pains, the terrifying condition known as angina. For some, it was so agonizing that they couldn't lie down and had to sleep sitting up. Only a few could take long walks, and some couldn't even cross a room without excruciating pain. The fact is that some were walking dead men.

It was, no doubt, because they had completely run out of options that they agreed to the demanding conditions I set for entry into the trial cure that I had come to believe in.

What they had to give up, I explained, would not be easy for any American accustomed to a diet flush with deep-fried fast foods, thick steaks, and rich dairy products. But if they were prepared to join me in a diet not unlike the one followed by two-thirds of the world's population, I held out the likelihood that we could overturn the death sentences that had been delivered to them by their physicians. In the process, we could demonstrate that the leading killer of Americans, heart disease, was a paper tiger that could be defeated—and without the use of a surgeon's knife.

By now, most everyone is generally aware that what you eat has something to do with whether or not you will develop heart disease. Back when my study began, this wasn't at all established. But also out of a personal sense of threat—everyone in my family had died early—I had begun looking for some alternative fate and had come up with the idea of low-fat, plant-based nutrition. On the West Coast, unbeknownst to me, Dean Cornish had started down the same path with several earlier published studies showing the benefits of lifestyle change. There we were, on opposite sides of the continent, not knowing nor having heard of each other at the time.

Almost all of those who came to me, who had been told there was little hope, today—twenty years later—are alive, their arterial diseases receded. They stand as living proof of what is possible for you and anyone else who chooses to do what is necessary to become heart-attack–proof. And they gave me the invaluable gift of confidence as I went on to counsel and treat hundreds of additional patients.

This book is dedicated to those original patients—to the adventure we had together, pioneering this experiment in the treatment of coronary heart disease, and to the way they picked up their lives and found, in the course of pursuing an alternative diet and lifestyle, a resumption of the joy of living. It offers a simple, basic hopeful way for you to navigate your way into a long and rewarding life.

Let me tell you the story of my patients, of our research, and of what we have learned.

PART ONE

The Heart of the Matter

I

Eating to Live

"IT WAS A FRIDAY in November 1996. I had operated all day. I finished, said good-bye to my last patient, and got a very, very bad headache. It hit me in a flash. I had to sit down. A minute or two after that, the chest pain started. It radiated up my arm and shoulder and into my jaw."

These are the words of Joe Crowe, the doctor who succeeded me as chairman of the breast cancer task force at the Cleveland Clinic. He was having a heart attack. He was only forty-four years old. He had no family history of heart disease, was not overweight or diabetic, and did not have high blood pressure or a bad cholesterol count. In short, he was not the usual candidate for a heart attack. Nonetheless, he had been struck—and struck hard.

In this book, I tell Joe Crowe's story, along with those of many other patients I have treated over the past twenty years. My subject is coronary artery disease, its cause, and the revolutionary treatment, available to all, that can abolish it and that has saved Joe Crowe and many others. My message is clear and absolute: *coronary artery disease need not exist, and if it does, it need not progress.* It is my dream that one day we may entirely abolish heart disease, the scourge of the affluent, modern West, along with an impressive roster of other chronic illnesses.

Here are the facts. Coronary artery disease is the leading killer of men and women in Western civilization. In the United States alone, more than half a million people die of it every single year. Three times that number suffer known heart attacks. And approximately three million more have "silent" heart attacks, experiencing minimal symptoms and having no idea, until well after the damage is done, that they are in mortal danger. In the course of a lifetime, one out of every two American men and one out of every three American women will have some form of the disease.

The cost of this epidemic is enormous—greater, by far, than that of any other disease. The United States spends more than $250 billion a year on heart disease. That's about the same amount the nation spent on the first two and half years of its military venture in Iraq, and fully twice as much as the federal government allocates annually for all research and development—including R&D for defense and national security.[1]

But here is the truly shocking statistic: nearly all of that money is devoted to treating symptoms. It pays for cardiac drugs, for clot-dissolving medications, and for costly mechanical techniques that bypass clogged arteries or widen them with balloons, tiny rotating knives, lasers, and stents. All of these approaches carry significant risk of serious complications, including death. And even if they are successful, they provide only temporary relief from the symptoms. *They do nothing at all to cure the underlying disease or to prevent its development in other potential victims.*

I believe that we in the medical profession have taken the wrong course. It is as if we were simply standing by, watching millions of people march over a cliff, and then intervening in a desperate, last-minute attempt to save them once they have fallen over the edge. Instead, we should be teaching them how to avoid the chasm entirely, how to walk parallel to the precipice so that they will never fall at all.

I believe that coronary artery disease is preventable, and that even after it is under way, its progress can be stopped, its insidious effects reversed. I believe, and my work over the past twenty years has demonstrated, that all this can be accomplished without expensive mechanical intervention and with minimal use of drugs. The key lies in nutrition—specifically, in abandoning the toxic American diet and maintaining cholesterol levels well below those historically recommended by health policy experts.

The bottom line of the nutritional program I recommend is that it contains not a single item of any food known to cause or promote the development of vascular disease. I often ask patients to compare their coronary artery disease to a house fire. Your house is on fire because eating the wrong foods has given you heart disease. You are spraying gasoline on the fire by continuing to eat the very same foods that caused the disease in the first place.

I don't want my patients to pour a single thimbleful of gasoline on the fire. Stopping the gasoline puts out the fire. Reforming the way you eat will end the heart disease.

Here are the rules of my program in their simplest form:

- You may not eat anything with a mother or a face (no meat, poultry, or fish).

- You cannot eat dairy products.

- You must not consume oil of any kind—not a drop. (Yes, you devotees of the Mediterranean Diet, that includes olive oil, as I'll explain in Chapter 10.)

- Generally, you cannot eat nuts or avocados.

You *can* eat a wonderful variety of delicious, nutrient-dense foods:

- All vegetables except avocado. Leafy green vegetables, root vegetables, veggies that are red, green, purple, orange, and yellow and everything in between.

- All legumes—beans, peas, and lentils of all varieties.

- All whole grains and products, such as bread and pasta, that are made from them—as long as they do not contain added fats.

- All fruits.

It works. In the first continuous twelve-year study of the effects of nutrition in severely ill patients, which I will describe in this book, those who complied with my program achieved total arrest of clinical progression and significant selective reversal of coronary artery disease. In fully compliant patients, we have seen angina disappear in a few weeks and abnormal stress test results return to normal.

And consider the case of Joe Crowe. After his heart attack in 1996, tests showed that the entire lower third of his left anterior descending coronary artery—the vessel leading to the front of the heart and nicknamed, for obvious reasons, "the widowmaker"—was significantly diseased. His coronary artery anatomy excluded him as a candidate for surgical bypass, angioplasty, or stents, and at such a young age, with a wife and three small children, Dr. Crowe was understandably disconsolate and depressed. Since he already exercised, did not use tobacco, and had a relatively low cholesterol count of 156 milligrams per deciliter (mg/dL), there seemed to be nothing he could modify, no obvious reforms in lifestyle that might halt the disease.

Joe was aware of my interest in coronary disease. About two weeks after his heart attack, he and his wife, Mary Lind, came to dinner at our house and I had a chance to share the full details of my research. Both Joe and Mary Lind immediately grasped the implications for Joe of a plant-based diet. All at once, instead of having no options, they were empowered. In Mary Lind's words, "It was our own personal disaster, and suddenly there was something small we could do." Immediately, Joe embarked on my nutrition program, refusing to take any cholesterol-lowering drugs, and he redefined the word *commitment*. He stuck to the plan rigorously, eventually reducing his total blood cholesterol count to just 89 mg/dL and cutting his LDL, or "bad" cholesterol, from 98 mg/dL to 38 mg/dL.

About two and a half years after Joe adopted a strict plant-based diet, there came a point when he was exceptionally busy professionally, under considerable stress, and he noted a return of some discomfort in his chest. His cardiologists, worried about the recurrence of angina, asked for more tests to see what was going on.

On the day of his follow-up angiogram, I went to Dr. Crowe's office after work. After we greeted each other, I thought I saw moisture in his eyes. "Is everything OK?" I asked.

"You saved my life," he declared. "It's gone! It's not there anymore! Something lethal is gone! My follow-up angiogram was normal."

Nearly ten years later, Mary Lind recalled that they had wondered, that first evening at our house, "how the Esselstyns did it"—how we had managed to completely change the way we eat. "Now it's part of our family," she says. "We've eaten the same things for a long time, and I'm on autopilot."

Later, when I asked Joe what made him decide to change, he responded very simply. "We believed you," he said, and added, "since I had nothing else, the diet came first. If I had had bypass surgery, diet would not have been first. The diet set us on another path, empowered to do something we knew we could do."

Joe Crowe's angiograms—both the original, taken after the heart attack, and the follow-up, two and a half years later—are shown in Figure 1 (see insert). It is the most complete resolution of coronary artery disease I have seen, graphic proof of the power of plant-based nutrition to enable the body to heal itself.

The dietary changes that have helped my patients over the past twenty years can help you, too. They can actually make you immune to heart attacks. And there is considerable evidence that they have benefits far beyond coronary artery disease. If you eat to save your heart, you eat to save yourself from other diseases of nutritional extravagance: from strokes, hypertension, obesity, osteoporosis, adult-onset diabetes, and possibly senile mental impairment, as well. You gain protection from a host of other ailments that have been linked to dietary factors, including impotence and cancers of the breast, prostate, colon, rectum, uterus, and ovaries. And if you are eating for good health in this way, here's a side benefit you might not have expected: *for the rest of your life, you will never again have to count calories or worry about your weight.*

An increasing number of doctors are aware that diet plays a crucial role in health, and that nutritional changes such as those I recommend can have dramatic effects on the development and progression of disease. But for a number of reasons, current medical practice places little emphasis on primary and secondary prevention. For most physicians, nutrition is not of significant interest. It is not an essential pillar of medical education; each generation of medical students learns about a different set of pills and procedures, but receives almost no training in disease prevention. And in practice, doctors are not rewarded for educating patients about the merits of truly healthy lifestyles.

Over the past one hundred years, the mechanical treatment of disease has increasingly dominated the medical profession in the United States. Surgery is the prototype, and its dramatic progress—light-years removed from the cathartics, bloodletting, and amputations that dominated medicine in previous centuries—is nothing short of breathtaking. But surgery has serious flaws. It is expensive, painful, and frightening, often disabling and disfiguring, and too often merely a temporary stopgap against the disease it is intended to treat. It is a mechanical approach to a biological problem.

Perhaps no area of medicine better illustrates the mechanical approach to disease than cardiology and cardiac surgery. Consider: the United States contains just 5 percent of the global population, but every year, physicians in American hospitals perform more than 50 percent of all the angioplasties and bypass procedures in the entire world. One reason is that mechanical medicine is romantic and dramatic, a natural magnet for media attention. Remember the drama several years ago surrounding implants of artificial hearts?

Most of the recipients died within weeks of their surgery, and all lived their last days tethered to life-support machinery that, far from enhancing their quality of life, drastically reduced it. But no matter: the dramatic interventions engaged the national imagination for months on end.

All told, there has been little incentive for physicians to study alternate ways to manage disease, so the mechanical/procedural approach continues to dominate the profession even though it offers little to the unsuspecting millions about to become the next victims of disease. Modern hospitals offer almost nothing to enhance public health. They are cathedrals of sickness.

There are some signs of change. Physicians and researchers increasingly agree that lifestyle changes—controlling blood pressure, stopping smoking, reducing cholesterol, exercising, and modifying diets—are essential to overall health. It is hard to deny the evidence, mounting with every passing year, that people who have spent a lifetime consuming the typical American diet are in dire trouble. Dr. Lewis Kuller of the University of Pittsburgh recently reported the ten-year findings of the Cardiovascular Health Study, a project of the National Heart, Lung, and Blood Institute. His conclusion is startling: "All males over 65 years of age, exposed to a traditional Western lifestyle, have cardiovascular disease and should be treated as such."[2]

Even interventional cardiologists are beginning to question the rationale of their procedures. In 1999, cardiologist David Waters of the University of California performed a study that compared the results of angioplasty—in which a balloon is inserted into a coronary artery to widen the vessel and improve blood flow—with the use of drugs to aggressively reduce serum cholesterol levels. There was no disputing the outcome. The patients who had the drug treatment to lower cholesterol had fewer hospitalizations for chest pain and fewer heart attacks than those who underwent angioplasty and standard postoperative care.[3]

The larger lesson of that study is that systemic treatment of disease through aggressive reduction of cholesterol is clearly superior to selective intervention at a single site where an artery has been clogged and narrowed. And it caused considerable uproar among cardiologists. As Dr. Waters observes, "There is a tradition in cardiology that doesn't want to hear that."

Why? Money! For many years, I resisted that conclusion, but the weight of the evidence is overwhelming. Interventional cardiologists earn hundreds of thousands of dollars annually, and particularly busy ones make millions. In addition, cardiology procedures generate huge revenues for hospitals. And the insurance industry supports the mechanical/procedural approach to vascular disease. It is far easier to document and quantify procedures for reimbursement than it is to document and quantify lifestyle changes that prevent the need for such procedures in the first place.

As a physician, I am embarrassed by my profession's lack of interest in healthier lifestyles. We need to change the way we approach chronic disease.

The work I will describe in the following chapters confirms that sustained nutrition changes and, when necessary, low doses of cholesterol-reducing medication will offer maximum protection from vascular disease. Anyone who follows the program faithfully will almost certainly see no further progression of disease, and will very likely find that it selectively regresses. And the corollary, overwhelmingly supported by global population studies, is that persons without the disease who adopt these same dietary changes will never develop heart disease.

Cardiologists who have seen my peer-reviewed data often concede that coronary artery disease may be arrested and reversed through changes in diet and lifestyle, but then add that they don't believe their patients would follow such "radical" nutritional changes.

But the truth is that there is nothing radical about my nutrition plan. It's about as mainstream as you can get. For 4 billion of the world's 5.5 billion people, the nutrition program I recommend is standard fare, and heart disease and many other chronic ailments are almost unknown. The word *radical* better describes the typical American diet, which guarantees that millions will perish from withering vascular systems. And in my experience, patients who realize that they have a clear choice—between invasive surgery that will do nothing to cure their underlying disease and nutritional changes that will arrest and reverse the disease and improve the quality of their lives—willingly adopt the dietary changes.

One of my patients, Jerry Murphy, came to me at the age of sixty-seven after his cardiologist recommended open heart surgery, something he was determined to avoid. "No male Murphy has ever lived beyond sixty-seven," he announced. "What are you going to do about that?" I responded that the real question was what *he* was going to do about it, albeit with my help. Now in his mid-eighties—well past the sixty-seven-year life expectancy for male Murphys—Jerry Murphy thinks my nutrition program represents a more natural way of eating, a return to healthier ways of the past. "It made sense to me," he says, citing his Irish ancestors, who may have killed the fatted calf once a year, but who subsisted primarily on a low-fat, plant-based diet.

Each of us has friends, family, and acquaintances who are the victims of coronary disease. These people are often vigorous, in the prime of life, when they are struck down by a heart attack. If they survive, they are rarely the same again, always fearful of another attack or the onset of some complication. Those close to them share similar concerns. But the truth is that this disease need never occur at all. For the great majority of this planet's population—the 4 billion who do not participate in the Western lifestyle—it simply does not exist.

I have an ambitious goal: to annihilate heart disease—to abolish it once and for all. Your arteries at the age of ninety ought to work as efficiently as they did when you were nine. My nutritional program is strict, and allows no shortcuts. I am uncompromising. I am authoritative. But as I always tell my patients, I am a caring presence. I want to see people succeed, and if they share my vision, they will.

If you do what I ask, your disease is history. Rather than detour around it, squish it with a balloon or brace it open with a wire bracket—either of which is just a temporary angina-relieving procedure—my program can prevent disease altogether, or stop it in its tracks. All the interventional procedures carry considerable risk of morbidity, including new heart attacks, strokes, infections, and, for some, an inevitable loss of cognition. Mine carries none. And the benefits of intervention erode with the passage of time; eventually, you have to have another angioplasty, another bypass procedure, another stent. By contrast, the benefits of my program actually grow with time. The longer you follow it, the healthier you will be.

A few years ago, I was on a cruise ship giving a presentation about my nutrition program and its dramatic results in patients with severe coronary artery disease. Toward the end a man in a straw hat approached me, and near tears, with audible anger in his voice, said, "I've been doing everything my doctor told me to, and now I have to have a second bypass. I can't believe no one told me there was another option!"

That's the point of this book: to tell the world what I have learned.

2

"Someday We'll Have to Get Smarter"

When I returned in 1968 from duty as an Army surgeon in Vietnam, I was offered a position in the Department of General Surgery at the Cleveland Clinic in Cleveland, Ohio. My major specialties were thyroid, parathyroid, gastrointestinal, and breast surgery, but I was always interested in vascular medicine, and made a point of taking extra training in the subject.

Medicine ran in the family. My father, Caldwell B. Esselstyn, was a distinguished physician, a great innovator in group practice in upstate New York. It was his idea to bring to a rural county all the best in medicine—from dentistry and psychiatry to obstetrics-gynecology and pediatrics—using a rotating roster of specialists. My father-in-law, the late Dr. George Crile, Jr., had been a breast cancer pioneer at the Cleveland Clinic, which had been founded by his father. When he started practicing medicine, radical mastectomies were still the order of the day; it was his vision that the surgery did not always have to be so extensive, and he devoted much of his professional life to developing less radical operations.

But something besides medicine also ran in the family. Both my father and my father-in-law were living examples of the toxic

American diet. Between them, they had diabetes; strokes; prostate, colon, and lung cancer; and coronary artery disease. About three years before my father died of heart disease in 1975, he said something that has stayed with me ever since: "Someday, we're just going to have to get smarter about showing people how to live healthier lives."

Everything in my professional experience underscored the importance of that declaration. Despite my father-in-law's pioneering work, for example, by the time I arrived at the Cleveland Clinic, many women were still losing breasts or being disfigured by surgery for breast cancer. And although I enjoyed my work as a surgeon—I take great pride in surgery that is well performed, that achieves a positive result, and relieves suffering—I was increasingly disillusioned by what I was *not* doing: never curing the underlying disease, never doing anything to help prevent it in the next victim. I was distressed by the general lack of interest among physicians in preventing cancer and heart disease, rather than intervening mechanically once they had struck.

I began reading a great deal of medical literature, with a particular emphasis on epidemiology. There was a beautiful simplicity to the evidence. You looked at a map of the world, and almost all the chronic ailments like coronary disease were crowded into the western countries. Then there were all these other countries, especially in Asia and Africa, where those diseases hardly showed up at all.

For example, women in the United States were twenty times more likely than women in Kenya to develop breast cancer.[1] And in the early 1950s, breast cancer was almost unknown in Japan (later, the rates began to rise as the Japanese adopted lifestyles—and eating habits—more like those of affluent Westerners). A close look at the cultures with low rates of breast cancer showed an obvious common denominator: a low intake of dietary fat and correspondingly low cholesterol levels. The same was true for cancers of the colon, prostate, and ovary, and for diabetes and obesity.[2]

The more I read, the more convinced I became that the connection between nutrition and disease was critical. The correlation seemed most vivid in coronary artery disease, the leading killer of men and women in the United States. It has become clearer in the past decade or so, but even twenty years ago, the general reading was that the connection between cholesterol and heart disease was paramount. The epidemiological evidence seemed incontrovertible. In those parts of the world where coronary artery disease is rare, diets are low in fat and serum cholesterol levels are consistently below 150 mg/dL. In the United States, where vascular disease is the leading killer, the average citizen eats sixty-five pounds of fat per year—consuming *two tons* of suet by the age of sixty—and average cholesterol levels hover around 200 mg/dL.[3]

Autopsies of soldiers during the Korean and Vietnam wars showed the effects of America's artery-clogging diet even on the very young. The arteries of Asian soldiers were largely clean, free of fatty deposits. But almost 80 percent of American battlefield casualties showed gross evidence of coronary artery disease—clogging and damage that, had the soldiers lived, would have grown worse with every passing decade.[4] What's more, in recent years, researchers have observed that as residents of areas with a low incidence of cardiovascular disease begin to adopt a more Western style of life and diet, the incidence of disease—especially coronary disease—rises dramatically.

It may be years before we understand each step and every nuance of the process by which dietary fat and cholesterol destroy coronary arteries. But we are well aware of the general outlines. Simply stated, just as you need stone to build a stone wall, you need a specific level of fat and cholesterol in your bloodstream to narrow and clog your arteries with atherosclerosis.

When the cholesterol carried in the bloodstream reaches unsafe levels—levels I will discuss in Chapter 4—fat and cholesterol are deposited on the linings of the blood vessels. These deposits are called plaques. Old plaques may contain scar tissue and calcium and can steadily enlarge, severely narrowing and sometimes blocking the arteries. A significantly narrowed artery cannot supply the heart muscle with adequate blood. Heart muscle deprived of normal blood supply causes chest pain, or angina (see Figure 2 in insert).

Most people think that it is the vessel's finally closing off, completely blocked by a large old plaque, that causes a heart attack, or myocardial infarction. Wrong. That process actually accounts for only about 12 percent of deaths from heart attacks. The most recent scientific evidence shows that most heart attacks are caused by younger fatty plaques—plaques too small to cause the overt symptoms that ordinarily bring on mechanical interventions like angioplasty.

Here's what happens: the lining that covers such plaques ruptures, and the fatty deposits inside leach out into the bloodstream. The body responds by rushing its clotting forces to repair the injury. When the clotting process succeeds, the entire artery may clot and close, thus completely depriving an area of heart muscle of its blood supply, causing it to die (see Figure 3 in insert).

If a person survives such an attack, the dead portion of heart muscle scars. Multiple heart attacks and widespread scarring weaken the heart, sometimes causing it to fail, a condition called congestive heart failure. If a heart attack is extensive, if it disrupts rhythmical contraction, or if congestive heart failure is prolonged, the victim may die.

My research shows that this entire process is preventable—and that through nutrition (plus, in some cases, low doses of cholesterol-lowering drugs) the risk of heart attack and heart failure can be eliminated. Scientists and physicians have been slow to recognize the connection between nutrition and coronary disease. In part, that's because the development of the disease is not like, say, a bee sting, in which the relationship between cause and effect is quite obvious. It may require decades of self-injury from a high-fat diet before clinical symptoms develop.

But truth to tell, when scientists peer too deeply into the most minute details of a problem, they sometimes miss the obvious solution. Sometimes, intuition and logic point strongly to an answer that has not yet been proven through the scientific method. There are some classic examples in medical history. In the mid–nineteenth century, for instance, an English physician named John Snow removed the handle from the Broad Street pump in London because he was convinced that somehow the shared water was causing a devastating cholera epidemic. He was right. It was many decades later that science identified the waterborne organism that causes cholera, but Dr. Snow intuited what the problem was, and he saved the town.

Similarly, we do not know even today precisely how insulin does its job of escorting blood sugar into the body's cells to be converted to energy. Nevertheless, doctors have been using insulin to save the lives of diabetics for more than eighty years. We know the connection is crucial even though we do not understand exactly how.

By the late 1970s, I was certain that there was a strong connection between nutrition and many diseases. The connection with heart disease seemed most obvious. First, there was the compelling fact that in nations where blood levels of cholesterol were customarily below 150 mg/dL, coronary artery disease was rare, while in places where the levels were higher, so was the incidence of heart disease. In addition, the earliest scientific studies—which have been consistently confirmed by the most recent research—showed that a diet high in fat and cholesterol causes coronary artery disease in animals and humans.

My own logic and intuition strongly suggested that the converse might also be true: reducing fat in the diet might make coronary artery disease cease to progress—and even partially reverse. In fact, this had been demonstrated in monkeys. They had acquired the disease after being fed a diet deliberately loaded with fat; when the dietary fat was reduced, their disease had reversed.[5] There was no doubt in my mind that further research into the nutrition-disease connection was well worth the effort.

Our local dietitians were skeptical about my theory, and several senior cardiologists at the Cleveland Clinic did not believe there was a connection between diet and coronary disease. Nonetheless, I pursued my studies.

Then, in April 1984, I had a personal epiphany—and in effect became the first subject of my own experiment. I was with my wife, Ann, at a meeting of the Eastern Surgical Society in New Haven, Connecticut. It was pouring rain. I was wet and uncomfortable—thoroughly disgusted with the day. And then a waitress served me a plate containing a huge, bloody slice of roast beef. Suddenly, I was repelled by the meat along with everything else. At that moment, I gave it all up—decided never to consume meat again.

Ann ate every bite of that meal in New Haven. But it was not long before she, too, adopted a plant-based diet. Her mother had died of breast cancer at the age of fifty-two. And one day, at an aunt's house, just as lunch was about to begin at the aunt's eighty-fifth birthday party, Ann's sister called. She, too, had been diagnosed with breast cancer, at the age of forty-eight. Ann sat down and didn't eat a bit of that lunch. And she joined me in my dietary experiment.

Between April and June 1984, my cholesterol level fell from 185 mg/dL to 155. This still was not acceptable. Next, I omitted from my diet every possible source of oil and dairy fat (milk, butter, ice cream, cheese). Before long, my blood cholesterol was 119 mg/dL—without the use of any cholesterol-lowering medication. This was especially reassuring, since my late father, who had his first heart attack at age forty-three, had a total cholesterol as high as 300 mg/dL.

I was convinced that I could help others achieve similar results, and that the effects on their health would be nothing short of dramatic.

3

Seeking the Cure

IN 1985, William Sheldon, chief of the Department of Cardiology at the Cleveland Clinic, graciously granted my request to attend a departmental meeting. I asked the cardiologists to refer patients with advanced coronary artery disease to participate in a study. My goal: to use plant-based nutrition to reduce the patients' cholesterol levels to below 150 mg/dL—the level seen in cultures where the disease is virtually nonexistent—and to see what effect it had on their health.

My original intent was to have one group of patients eating a very-low-fat diet and another receiving standard cardiac care, and then to compare how the two groups had fared after three years. This approach, due to a lack of funding, was not practical. Nevertheless, I believed that proceeding without a control group for comparison could yield significant findings. And since I was not using any new medicines or procedures, my experiment—which represented, essentially, a study of the practice of medicine—was approved by the clinic's internal review board. What was different about this experiment was that for my patients, the standard cardiac diet would be unacceptable. I was going to see to it that they followed a truly low-fat, plant-based diet.

The first patient entered the program in October 1985, and by 1988, the cardiologists at the Cleveland Clinic had referred twenty-four patients to me. All were suffering from advanced coronary artery disease, and most were debilitated by angina and other symptoms. The majority had undergone one or two failed bypasses or angioplasty and either had refused further traditional treatment or were ineligible for it. None smoked, none were hypertensive.

The group included twenty-three men and one woman. They agreed to follow a plant-based diet. (It turned out that between 9 and 12 percent of the calories they consumed on that diet were derived from fat.) I asked them to eliminate from their diet almost all dairy products (in the beginning, I allowed them to have skim milk and nonfat yogurt, but have since eliminated all dairy products because of the potential tumor-causing properties of caseine[1] and the contribution of animal protein to the process of atherosclerosis), all oil and all fish, fowl, and meat. I encouraged them to eat grains, legumes, lentils, vegetables, and fruit. I asked them to keep daily food diaries listing everything they consumed, recommended that they take a daily multivitamin, and suggested that they moderate their consumption of alcohol and caffeine. And each participant received a prescription for a cholesterol-lowering drug. In the beginning, the drug was usually cholestyramine. In 1987, when the first of the statins, lovastatin, became available, that became our drug of choice.[2]

The most frequent objection I had heard to my ideas about nutrition—and it's the same objection I hear to this very day—was that patients would never comply with such major changes in their diet. So I was determined to give them all the support I possibly could. Years before, I'd heard the pioneering physician J. Engelbert Dunphy quoted as saying that cancer patients are not afraid of suffering or dying, but are afraid of being abandoned. That became my mantra with my study group: I would never allow them to feel abandoned.

From the very start, I made it a point to be integrally involved in each participant's treatment. It began with an initial interview of forty-five to sixty minutes with each patient and his or her spouse. We reviewed medical history, cultural variations in heart disease, research findings in human and animal studies, and the various therapeutic options that were available. I wanted everyone to understand just exactly what I was recommending—and why.

Then, every two weeks, I met each patient in my office to go over every morsel of food he or she had eaten in the previous fortnight. I checked blood pressure and weight and had blood cholesterol drawn and analyzed. During the first year of the study, I called each patient the night of the tests to report the results and make any adjustments in nutrition or medication that seemed necessary.

It is highly unusual for a physician to see a patient every two weeks for more than five years, but it seemed absolutely crucial to me that I provide all the support and focus for them that I possibly could. They had to recognize that even though an angioplasty or bypass operation might have failed them, they could achieve control over their own disease by totally eliminating the dietary fats that had been killing them in the first place.

I did not require participants in the study to commit to any extra measures, such as exercise or meditation. There are several reasons for that. For one, it was my observation that in those cultures where coronary disease does not exist, it was diet and low cholesterol, not exercise habits or personal tranquillity, that were responsible for warding it off. For another, I think every human being has just so many personal behavior modification units available—that is, if you're asked to change too much, you will eventually balk!—and I was already asking a great deal of my patients. It was imperative that they focus all their capacity for changing their behavior on modifying their diets and reducing cholesterol levels in order to arrest and control their disease. So even though relaxation, meditation, and regular exercise have demonstrable health benefits, for this program, they remained entirely optional.

. . .

It was clear almost from the beginning that six patients just did not grasp what we were trying to accomplish, and that they would not comply with the experiment. So by mutual agreement, I returned them to their cardiologists for standard care with the understanding that I would periodically check to see how they were doing. But the rest stuck with the program. They ranged in age from forty-three to sixty-seven years old. And they represented a spectrum of the community. They were factory workers, teachers, office employees, company executives.

Each approached the program in his or her own way. Jerry Murphy, the one who had challenged me ("No male Murphy has ever lived beyond sixty-seven"), says he found it relatively easy to follow the rules, although his daughter, Rita, describes the new diet he adopted as "a life-changing event" for the rest of the family, whose members had to learn to cook and eat in an entirely new way.

Some felt they simply had no choice but to try what I recommended. Don Felton, for example, was fifty-four when he came to me. He had been suffering from heart problems since the age of twenty-seven, when he first experienced severe chest pain. "The doctors fluffed it off," he says, and one even said that the problem was "all in his head"—a suggestion that infuriated him.

Three years later, still plagued by chronic pain, he underwent two days of tests and a catheterization at his local hospital. When he got the results, the news was not good. "People with the severity of disease you have average about a year," the cardiologist told him. Since the doctors were afraid to operate, they prescribed medication for the pain, and the hospital dietician actually advised him to consume a stick of corn oil margarine every day—a prescription based on some study (we now know far better) that suggested corn oil was good for the heart and arteries! Don couldn't stomach the idea of eating a stick of margarine, so instead, he dutifully poured corn oil into a glass and drank it before he went to bed each night for several years.

By the time Don was forty-four, he was sicker than ever. Several times, he collapsed on hunting trips. His wife, Mackie, recalls that every time an ambulance went by, their son, who worked at a gas station not far from the Feltons' house, called home to see if it was carrying his father.

Eventually, Don had to quit his job as manager of an Ohio plant that manufactured hydraulic power units for airplane simulators. He went on disability. And finally, when he was forty-eight, he had bypass surgery. But within a few years, the veins used for the bypass closed. After a frightening episode of chest pain while on a hunting trip when he was fifty-four, Don's doctor said there was nothing more he could do. "But he wanted to offer me something," Don says, so he mentioned that a physician named Esselstyn was offering some kind of program. At that point, Don says, "I was willing to try anything. What did I have to lose?"

Similarly, Emil Huffgard had pretty much run out of choices by the time he came to see me. At the age of thirty-nine, he had suffered a stroke. A few years later, he had bypass surgery—and then, in rapid succession, three more strokes. He was in dreadful shape, relying on nitroglycerin to get him through days of terribly constricted activity. "Any walking brought on the angina," says Emil. "I could shower, shave, read the paper. And I was pretty good at sitting down." Surgery was out of the question—likely to kill him, the cardiologist explained. After years of agony, the cardiologist told Emil about Dr. Esselstyn, and suggested that he have a talk with me.

His back was against the wall. There was no mechanical intervention he could have. He was gobbling nitro all day to stave off the angina, and couldn't even lie down flat to sleep. Every day, his wife, Margie, had to cover his thorax and abdomen with nitroglycerin paste, which she then covered with plastic wrap to protect his clothes, just so that Emil could perform the most basic tasks of taking care of himself without suffering incapacitating pain. She had actually advised their daughter to move up her wedding date if she wanted her father to walk her down the aisle—advice their daughter took. When he joined my program, with a cholesterol count of 307, Emil was desperate.

So was Anthony Yen. He had been raised in China before the Communist takeover, a member of one of that nation's wealthiest families. While growing up, he ate a relatively healthy diet that contained very little meat and oil. But when he came to the United States to attend the Massachusetts Institute of Technology, everything changed. It was not long before he was positively bingeing on the artery-clogging American diet: "lots of hamburgers and lots of cheeseburgers, a lot of spaghetti and meatballs." For breakfast, he routinely ate bacon and eggs. And he came to love fried food—especially French fries.

Anthony graduated from MIT, and after serving an apprenticeship in corporate America, he started his own international business, with headquarters in Cleveland. Through his family's many contacts in Korea, Japan, Taiwan, and Hong Kong, he set up operations in Southeast Asia to develop metalworking industries. He traveled a great deal, and whether at home or on the road, he continued to be—his own description—a "glutton." "I was gaining weight," he says, "but since I had my clothes tailor-made in Hong Kong, I'd have a suit made every trip, and didn't really notice that the old suits didn't fit."

On New Year's Eve, 1987, when Anthony was fifty-eight, he and his wife, Joseanne, booked a two-day holiday package deal at a hotel, which included dinner and dancing. Although it was the sort of activity he ordinarily loved, he felt awful—tired, overheated, and weak. And he felt pressure on his chest. The next morning, he says, he felt what he describes as a "boom" in his chest, and his wife insisted that he go to the Cleveland Clinic for a checkup.

After he underwent a stress test—quickly aborted when it showed abnormalities—and an angiogram, Anthony had quintuple bypass surgery. He went home to recuperate, but was utterly terrified, frightened even of moving, and grew deeply depressed. The family made an appointment with a psychologist. "I blamed myself for what I had done to myself," Anthony recalls. "I wanted to know what caused my disease, and how do I stop it." After listening to his story, the psychologist told him there was a doctor in the building named Esselstyn whose program might be of interest to him.

When Anthony informed his cardiologist that he was going to see me, the cardiologist objected. "Esselstyn is *not* a cardiologist," he declared. "If you go to him, don't come back to see me." Anthony was furious. "I wanted to get to the cause, and the doctor was so negative. So I fired the cardiologist, and went to Dr. Esselstyn on my own." As Joseanne explains, "He had *no hope*. He was willing to do anything."

Not everyone was quite so open to my message. Take Evelyn Oswick, for example—the group's only woman. She had been fifty-three when she suffered the first signs of heart trouble. She and her husband, Hank, had delivered their daughter to college, and were carrying a light chair up the stairs to the dormitory's second floor when Evelyn suddenly felt breathless. "It was scary, because my mother had had a heart condition and my brother had died of a heart attack in his early fifties," she says. So she went to the Cleveland Clinic for a checkup. She was pedaling away on a bicycle used for stress tests, and feeling no pain. But suddenly the doctor started shouting: "You're having a heart attack! You're having a heart attack!" The very next day, she had a triple bypass.

For the next five years, Evelyn, who taught speech and communication at John Carroll University in Cleveland, continued to eat all the food she loved. But there came a time, as she recalls, when she realized she just didn't feel well. "I had no pains scaring me, but there was a little pain in my left arm." The discomfort continued, and finally, Evelyn decided to go to the clinic. Hank was out of town on business, so she asked her daughter to go with her. As she lay on the examining table, the doctor started yelling, "She's having a heart attack!" ("Those words, once again!" Evelyn exclaims.) They rushed her to an angiography room, where she suddenly felt quite breathless.

The doctors told Evelyn that there was nothing they could do. Surgery, they said, was out of the question. Her primary doctor did mention a physician at the clinic who was doing a study, and he called me in to see her. I told her about the nutrition program.

Evelyn clearly remembers her reaction: "*No way!* I was very adamant. I loved my chocolate candy, cake, pie, and banana splits. I liked all the bad things. All the things I liked, he said I couldn't have. There was *no way* I would do that."

After she spent a few days in the hospital, Evelyn's doctor said, "Go home. Find a rocker." Evelyn remembers her response: "I should find a rocking chair and rock until the day I die?" The doctor replied, kindly enough, "That's what I mean." As Evelyn saw it, he had told her to go home and wait to die.

So she did. And for several days, she and Hank talked over the situation. The more they talked, the more Evelyn began to reexamine her attitude. "I was fifty-eight," she recalls. "Hank and I were at the peak of our lives. We had nothing when we started. Now we had everything we had ever wanted. There was no way I was going to die and have Hank marry someone else. Would I die and leave this money for another woman? No way. Then Hank laughed, and I laughed, and I said, 'I think we'll go to see Dr. Esselstyn.'"

When Evelyn walked into my office, I told her the truth: after our interview in the hospital, I never thought I would see her again. I was delighted that I turned out to be wrong.

Jim Trusso, the youngest of the group, was also a surprise. At first, I was pretty sure he wouldn't stick with the program. He'd been thirty-four when he had his first heart attack. He was washing his car one Sunday and suddenly felt breathless and congested. His self-diagnosis was that he was suffering a bronchitis attack. The next day, he was in a meeting at the elementary school where he was the principal, and he felt pressure in his chest. He decided to go to the hospital for some medicine to combat the "bronchitis."

He suspected, before anyone told him, that something was seriously wrong. "Electrocardiograms were taken on a roll of tape back then," Jim recalls. "A cute little nurse walked out without tearing the tape, and it was trailing behind her, unraveling out of the emergency room door." Sure enough, it turned out, the electrocardiogram indicated that Jim needed a catheterization.

During that procedure, the doctors discovered that he had sustained a massive heart attack, and they reported that there was too much muscle damage to allow surgery. No one told Jim the whole story at the time, but one of the physicians did tell Jim's wife, Sue, that he didn't have long to live and she might have to go back to work as a teacher to support their two small children.

A month later, Jim felt considerably better. He underwent a second catheterization. This time, the doctor said the muscle damage was not as great as they originally had feared, and declared him a prime candidate for bypass surgery.

After his surgery, Jim did very well—until the day, eight years later, when his chest pain suddenly returned. An evaluation convinced his doctors that he needed surgery once again. A second bypass.

Sue remembers wondering what on earth they were doing wrong. Then Jim heard of me from a former patient of mine who was painting Jim's condominium. When Jim informed his cardiologist that he wanted to see Dr. Esselstyn, the cardiologist bet him a steak dinner that he couldn't get his cholesterol below its level at the time—a frightening 305 mg/dL.

At first, I thought Jim was something of a wise guy, not entirely serious about the enterprise before us. We always seemed to be at loggerheads. He was constantly challenging me. What would he do at restaurants? While traveling? How could he possibly eat this food? He had always hated fruits and vegetables. "Big Macs, French fries, milk shakes were favorite foods," he readily admits. "My favorite thing was chocolate."

From the start, Jim made it sound as if what I asked him to do was absurd, a constant inconvenience. He deeply treasured the food that had gotten him in trouble. But he was an intelligent person, and what finally won him over was the logic of the program. We were trying to follow the nutritional example of countries where disease was nonexistent. To an educator, a man blessed with a supremely logical mind, it made sense.

It also made sense to Jack Robinson. Jack's father had died of heart disease while in his forties, and all three of Jack's brothers died of heart disease in their fifties. Jack was approaching that age in 1988, when he had an angiogram at the Cleveland Clinic. It showed multiple blockages of his coronary arteries. "They marched what seemed like eighty doctors through my room, insisting that I have bypass surgery," Jack says. But he adamantly refused, recalling the serious complications one of his brothers had experienced during a bypass operation. Unable to budge him, Jack says, "they suggested I consider seeing Dr. Esselstyn."

During counseling, Jack listened intently and fully understood what he had to do. He would have to follow the program at a distance. At the time, he was employed by General Tire in Akron. He told his local cardiologist, who was fully aware of the severity of disease shown by the Cleveland Clinic angiogram, how he planned to proceed. The cardiologist, despite serious misgivings, agreed to the plan.

In October 1985, we began our experiment with this diverse group of heart patients. Every three to four months, the entire group convened—usually at Ann's and my house—to share recipes, to compare how they were doing and emphasize the fact that they were not alone, and to reinforce their sense of commitment—to themselves and to each other. As a result, they developed lasting friendships and family connections. A strong sense of community and common purpose helped sustain them and encourage compliance.

I will tell you how things turned out for all these patients, and for others, as well. But first, you need to understand—just as I make sure my patients understand—the science behind what we were trying to accomplish.

4

A Primer on Heart Disease

THE GOAL OF MY STUDY was to use a combination of nutrition and cholesterol-reducing drugs to get the cholesterol levels of each and every one of my patients below 150 mg/dL and then to see what effect that reduction would have on their coronary artery disease.

I chose that particular target threshold for a number of reasons. For one, there was the clarion example of those parts of the world where cardiovascular disease is nearly nonexistent: in those areas, cholesterol levels are consistently below 150 mg/dL.[1] Cornell University professor emeritus Colin Campbell, an expert in biochemistry and nutrition, was the director of a twenty-year project that involved Cornell, Oxford University, and the Chinese Academy of Preventive Medicine—one of the most comprehensive studies of nutrition ever.[2] Among other things, the project found that the normal range of cholesterol among residents of rural China, where coronary artery disease is rarely seen, falls between 90 and 150 mg/dL. (Comparing those levels with levels in the United Kingdom, where cholesterol levels are far closer to those in the United States, Sir Richard Peto, an Oxford epidemiologist who worked with Dr. Campbell, couldn't resist commenting that when it comes to cholesterol, "There is no such thing as a normal Englishman.")

But there was also a growing body of work by physicians and scientists at home that underscored the evidence from abroad. Perhaps the most important was the Framingham Heart Study, the fifty-year project—run by the National Heart, Lung and Blood Institute, Boston University, and other academic collaborators—that has collected and analyzed medical data from several generations of residents of Framingham, Massachusetts. Dr. William Castelli, former director of the study, put it quite baldly: over all those years, no one in Framingham who maintained a cholesterol level lower than 150 mg/dL has had a heart attack.[3]

So why is your cholesterol level so important to your health? Let's take a look at some of the basics.

Cholesterol is a white, waxy substance that is not found in plants—only in animals. It is an essential component of the membrane that coats all our cells, and it is the basic ingredient of sex hormones. Our bodies need cholesterol, and they manufacture it on their own. We do not need to eat it. But we do, when we consume meat, poultry, fish, and other animal-based foods, such as dairy products and eggs. In doing so, we take on excess amounts of the substance. What's more, eating fat causes the body itself to manufacture excessive amounts of cholesterol, which explains why vegetarians who eat oil, butter, cheese, milk, ice cream, glazed doughnuts, and French pastry develop coronary disease despite their avoidance of meat.

Medicine subdivides cholesterol into two types. High-density lipoprotein, or HDL, is sometimes known as "good" cholesterol. Medical experts do not know precisely how, but it seems to offer some protection against heart attacks—by collecting excess cholesterol and carrying it away from the arteries to the liver, which can break it down and dispose of it. As total blood cholesterol rises, you need more and more of the HDL cholesterol to protect you against heart disease.

Low-density lipoprotein, or LDL, is "bad" cholesterol. When too much of it is present in the bloodstream, it tends to build up along artery walls, helping to form the plaques that narrow blood vessels and ultimately may clog them altogether.

The coronary arteries are the blood vessels that supply oxygen and nutrients to the muscle of the heart. They get their name from the Latin word for "crown" because they encircle the heart almost like a royal headpiece. They are relatively small, but exceedingly important: without the nourishment they bring to the incredibly efficient pump they serve, the heart becomes injured, begins to fail, and may die.

The innermost lining of all blood and lymph vessels and the heart is called the endothelium. Far more than a simple membrane, the endothelium is actually the body's single largest endocrine organ. If all the endothelial cells in your body were laid out flat, one cell thick, they would cover an area equal to two tennis courts.

Healthy arteries are strong and elastic, their linings smooth and unobstructed, allowing a free flow of blood. But when the levels of fats in the bloodstream become elevated, everything begins to change. Gradually, the endothelium, the white blood cells, and the platelets, the blood cells that cause clotting, all become sticky. Eventually, a white blood cell adheres to and eventually penetrates the endothelium, where it attempts to ingest the rising numbers of LDL cholesterol molecules that are being oxidized from the fatty diet. That white blood cell sends out a call for help to other white blood cells. More and more of them converge on the site, becoming engorged with bad cholesterol and eventually forming a bubble of fatty pus—an atheroma, or "plaque," the chief characteristic of atherosclerosis.

Old plaques contain scar tissue and calcium. As they enlarge, they severely narrow and sometimes block the arteries (see Figure 4 in insert). A significantly narrowed artery cannot give the heart muscle a normal blood supply, and the heart muscle, thus deprived, causes chest pain, or angina. In some cases, the coronary arteries actually perform their own bypasses, growing extra branches—called "collaterals"—that go around the narrowed vessels.

However, it is not the old, larger plaques that put you most at risk for heart attacks. The most recent scientific evidence indicates that most heart attacks occur when younger and smaller fatty plaques rupture their outer lining, or cap, and bleed into the coronary artery.

As the plaque is formed, a fibrous cap develops at its roof, which is covered by a single layer of endothelium about as thick as a cobweb. For a while, thus protected, plaques lie quietly in place, doing little perceptible harm to the artery's owner. But an insidious process is nonetheless under way. The white blood cells that raced to the rescue, now engorged with oxidized LDL cholesterol, are called "foam cells," and begin to manufacture chemical substances that erode the cap of the plaque. The cap weakens to the thickness of a cobweb. And eventually, the shearing force of blood flowing over the weakened cap may cause it to rupture.

This is catastrophic. Plaque content or pus now oozes into the flowing bloodstream, and that constitutes a thrombogenic event: nature wants to heal the rupture, and so platelets are activated. They try mightily to stop the invading garbage by clotting the rupture. Thus begins a lethal cascade. The clot is self-propagating, and within minutes, the entire artery may become blocked.

With no more blood flowing through the blocked artery, the heart muscle that was nourished by it begins to die. This is the definition of myocardial infarction, or heart attack. If the person survives this attack, the dead portion of heart muscle scars. Multiple heart attacks and widespread scarring weaken the heart, sometimes causing it to fail. That condition is known as congestive heart failure. If the heart attack is extensive, if it results in an abnormal rhythmical contraction, or if the congestive heart failure is prolonged, the person may die.

If the same process of plaque formation occurs in a noncoronary artery, it can be just as dangerous. Whatever tissue the artery supplies—it could be the leg muscles or even the brain—will not receive its full measure of blood. What's more, a piece of a plaque or a clot can break loose and be carried through the bloodstream, ultimately obstructing an artery far from its source.

Traditional cardiology has approached this disease primarily by relying on mechanical interventions. In angioplasty, for instance, a physician inserts a hollow tube into an artery in a leg or arm and guides it, using X-ray images, into the clogged coronary artery that is his target. A smaller catheter, with a deflated balloon at its tip, is then fed through the first. When it reaches the clogged area, the balloon is inflated—usually several times—to press the plaque against the artery wall, fracturing the plaque and the arterial wall, widening the vessel, and stripping away the delicate endothelial lining.

In recent years, the use of stents has become more common. A stent is a wire mesh tube that is inserted during angioplasty. When the balloon is inflated, the stent expands and locks into place inside the artery, holding it open after the balloon and catheter are withdrawn.

Bypass surgery is exactly what its name implies. The physician uses a short length of blood vessel from another part of the body to provide a way for blood to go around blockages in coronary arteries, much as a detour functions to route traffic around the congestion caused by an accident or by highway construction.

But as I have already argued, these interventions are aimed at alleviating the symptoms of coronary artery disease, not at curing the disease itself. And their results erode with the passage of time. Patients have second and third bypasses. Arteries widened with angioplasty tend to clog once again. Stents may have to be reopened because scar tissue reblocks the artery. The newer drug-eluting stents (coated with drugs to lessen the body's natural healing response to the injury caused by the stent's insertion) may also suddenly block after a few years because a clot forms where the endothelium was injured; the drug in the stent that prevents inflammation also inhibits the endothelium's capacity to heal.

We can do better. We can go right to the source of the disease. We can cut off the supply of fatty substances that accumulate in the arteries to such catastrophic effect.

We can go directly to the bottom line. This is it: *if you follow a plant-based nutrition program to reduce your total cholesterol level to below 150 mg/dL and the LDL level to less than 80 mg/dL, you cannot deposit fat and cholesterol into your coronary arteries.* Period.

And although some patients may need cholesterol-lowering drugs to help them achieve those safe, low cholesterol levels, drugs alone are not the answer. Nutrition is the real key to saving your life in the long term. Eating the right way not only will help reduce your cholesterol levels, but also can work additional wonders you may never have imagined.

5

Moderation Kills

A NUMBER OF YEARS AGO, when I was beginning my research project in coronary artery disease, a prominent local physician who disagreed with me announced that he believed in "dietary moderation" for his heart patients. Translation: I don't care if my heart patients eat *some* fat. That's a fairly common sentiment among my medical colleagues. But what are the facts?

In science, a review of many studies on the same subject is referred to as a meta-analysis. Such a review of studies on coronary artery disease was done in 1988, when researchers in Wisconsin analyzed ten clinical trials involving 4,347 patients.[1] Half of the patients had received cardiac rehabilitation, which generally consists of advice to lose weight, exercise, control high blood pressure, control diabetes, stop smoking, and eat less fat. The other half of the patients did not receive such assistance. The results: the "rehabilitated" group had slightly fewer fatal heart attacks than those who did not get the same advice. But the researchers found "no significant difference" between the two groups in the number of nonfatal heart attacks. In fact, the rehabilitated group suffered slightly more nonfatal attacks than those who made no lifestyle changes.

The reason is fairly simple. Those who moderately reduced their consumption of fat did manage to slow the rate of progression of their disease. But they did not completely arrest it, and as it progressed—even at its new, slower rate—it continued to take its toll.

In early 2006, a report published in *The Journal of the American Medical Association* resulted in national headlines suggesting that low-fat diets do not decrease health risks. The *JAMA* article was based on a study, part of the Women's Health Initiative of the National Institutes of Health, which followed nearly 49,000 women over eight years, and it found that those prescribed a "low-fat" diet turned out to have the same rates of heart attacks, strokes, and cancers of the breast and colon as those who ate whatever they wanted.[2]

Almost buried in the news reports about this latest, largest, most expensive study ever was this incredibly important fact: *the women who were supposedly consuming a low-fat diet were actually getting 29 percent of their daily calories from fat*. For those on the front lines of nutritional research, that is not "low fat" at all. It is three times the level—around 10 percent of daily caloric intake—that researchers like me recommend through plant-based nutrition.

The Women's Health Initiative study and the conclusions drawn from it bring to mind an analogy. Suppose researchers were studying the following question: does reducing vehicular speed save lives? They find that when a car strikes a stone wall at 90 miles an hour, all its occupants perish. The same result occurs when the car hits the wall at 80 mph—and at 70. Conclusion: reducing speed doesn't save lives. (Meanwhile, everyone ignores a small study showing that in a crash at 10 miles per hour, everyone survives.)

The Women's Health Initiative researchers were quoted as saying that their results "do not justify recommending low-fat diets to the public to reduce their heart disease and cancer risk." True, they certainly do not justify recommending diets containing 29 percent fat, the level currently endorsed in the U.S. Dietary Guidelines. But those of us who have been studying the matter already knew that. The Women's Health Initiative study simply confirms that the guidelines are wrong: we should be recommending diets far lower in fat than those featured in this research.

Over the years the meta-analyses, such as the one conducted by the Wisconsin researchers, have consistently shown that coronary patients who reduce their fat intake do somewhat better than those who do not. But almost always, the best outcome is a slowing of the rate of progression of disease in patients who receive treatment—not putting an absolute stop to it.

These results are not good enough. We should be aiming much higher: at arresting coronary artery disease altogether, even reversing its course. And the key to doing this, as my research demonstrates, is not simply reducing the amount of fat and cholesterol you ingest, but eliminating cholesterol and any fat beyond the natural, healthy amounts found in plants, from your diet. The key is plant-based nutrition.

Let's review what we know about the science. Heart disease, as I have already stressed, develops in susceptible persons when blood cholesterol levels rise higher than 150 mg/dL.[3] The converse is also true. A person who maintains blood cholesterol under 150 mg/dL for a lifetime will not develop coronary artery disease—even if he or she smokes, has a family history of coronary disease, suffers from hypertension, and is obese!

One case in point: the Papua Highlanders of New Guinea. These people are traditionally heavy smokers. Even nonsmokers among them breathe in lethal doses of secondhand smoke in communal hutches. Not surprisingly, the Papua Highlanders suffer many lung disorders, thanks to the smoking. But studies of those who live into their sixties and beyond have shown that despite the well-documented risk to heart health that is posed by smoking, they have no coronary artery disease.[4] They are protected by their diet, which consists almost entirely of nineteen separate varieties of sweet potatoes.

Nutrition impinges on cardiovascular health in several critical ways. The most obvious, of course, is that a diet high in fat and cholesterol causes blood lipid levels to rise, thus setting off the process of plaque formation.

But isn't "dietary moderation" enough to stop that process? If you cut back considerably on fat and cholesterol, shouldn't you be all right, as my colleague suggested? Surely, just a little bit wouldn't hurt.

Wrong! That's what you must remember every time you are confronted with that tempting tidbit topped with melted cheddar and bacon bits. Moderation kills. And to understand why, you have to understand something about metabolism and biochemistry.

Every segment of our bodies is comprised of cells, and every individual cell is protected by an outer coat. This cell membrane is almost unimaginably delicate—just one hundred-thousandth of a millimeter thick. Yet it is absolutely essential to the integrity and healthy functioning of the cell. And it is extremely vulnerable to injury.

Every mouthful of oils and animal products, including dairy foods, initiates an assault on these membranes and, therefore, on the cells they protect. These foods produce a cascade of free radicals in our bodies—especially harmful chemical substances that induce metabolic injuries from which there is only partial recovery. Year after year, the effects accumulate. And eventually, the cumulative cell injury is great enough to become obvious, to express itself as what physicians define as disease. Plants and grains do not induce the deadly cascade of free radicals. Even better, in fact, they carry an antidote. Unlike oils and animal products, they contain antioxidants, which help to neutralize the free radicals and also, recent research suggests, may provide considerable protection against cancers.

Among the body parts we injure every time we eat a typical American meal is the endothelium itself—the lining of the blood vessels and the heart—and the remarkable role it plays in maintaining healthy blood flow. The endothelial cells make nitric oxide, which is critical to preserving the tone and health of the blood vessels. Nitric oxide is a vasodilator: that is, it causes the vessels to dilate, or enlarge. When there is abundant nitric oxide in the bloodstream, it keeps blood flowing as if the vessels' surfaces were coated with the most slippery Teflon, eliminating the stickiness of vessels and blood cells that is caused by high lipid levels and that, in turn, leads to plaque formation.

There is mounting evidence of the critical importance of the endothelium. German researchers recently studied more than 500 patients diagnosed with coronary artery disease. They performed angiograms on the patients and also drew blood, quantifying the number of endothelial progenitor cells—the cells that restore and replace endothelium—in the bloodstream of each subject. Over the following twelve months, the researchers found that patients with the fewest endothelial progenitor cells fared most poorly. Those with the most cells did best of all.[5]

Dr. Robert Vogel, of the University of Maryland School of Medicine in Baltimore, has conducted some astonishing studies that demonstrate, among other things, what a toxic effect a single meal can have on the endothelium.[6] Dr. Vogel used ultrasound to measure the diameters of the brachial arteries of a group of students. Then he inflated blood pressure cuffs on the students' arms, stopping blood flow to their forearms for five minutes. After deflating the cuffs, he used the ultrasound to see how fast the arteries sprang back to their normal condition.

One group of students then ate a fast-food breakfast that contained 900 calories and 50 grams of fat. A second group ate 900-calorie breakfasts containing no fat at all. After they ate, Dr. Vogel again constricted their brachial arteries for five minutes and watched to see the result. It was dramatic. Among those who consumed no fat, there was simply no problem: their arteries bounced back to normal just as they had in the prebreakfast test. But the arteries of those who had eaten the fat-laden fast food took far longer to respond.

Why? The answer lies in the effect of fat on the endothelium's ability to produce nitric oxide. Dr. Vogel closely monitored endothelial function of subjects and found that two hours after eating a fatty meal there was a significant drop. It took nearly six hours, in fact, for endothelial function to get back to normal.

If a single meal can have such an impact on vascular health, imagine the damage done by three meals a day, seven days a week, 365 days a year—for decades.

But isn't it enough simply to reduce your cholesterol levels? Why insist upon a radical change in diet, if there are other ways to reach the cholesterol goals?

Recently, the *New England Journal of Medicine* reported on a study in which massive doses of cholesterol-lowering drugs were used to reduce total cholesterol well below 150 mg/dL. Three out of four of the heart patients involved seem to do very well under this regimen. But it was not a complete success. Even with their cholesterol levels satisfactorily reduced, one out of every four of the patients in the study sustained a new cardiovascular event or died within two and a half years of starting this treatment.[7]

I was struck by the fact that there were so many problems even though both total cholesterol and LDL levels in those patients were reduced well into the range I suggest and often below that. So I called the study's author, and discovered an extremely important variable: there had been no nutritional component to the study. When I asked what study participants had been eating, he replied, "It was a drug trial." They had continued to eat the same way they ate before the study began. That explains why so many patients failed.

Remember how I ask my patients to compare their disease to a house fire that they've been spraying with gasoline—and how I insist that in order to put it out, they must stop spraying it with fuel? That was the problem here. Despite profound cholesterol reduction with medication, the arterial plaque inflammation (the fire) and disease progression were inevitable because the patients were still ingesting the toxic American diet (the gasoline).

The patients in that study who died or whose disease progressed were subsequently tested for highly sensitive C-reactive protein, or HSCRP. This test measures the levels of a specific blood protein that increases with inflammation of the coronary arteries, and it is considered by many cardiologists to be even better than a standard cholesterol measurement at assessing your risk of heart attacks. All those patients who failed turned out to have elevated HSCRP levels.

There is a critical clue here to the overwhelming importance of nutrition. In my experience, fully compliant patients achieve normal levels of HSCRP within three to four weeks of adopting my plant-based nutrition program. The results are prompt, safe, and enduring.

Twenty years ago, when I started my research, our major focus was on reducing total blood cholesterol levels to below 150 mg/dL and cutting LDL levels to 80 mg/dL or less. But today, it is clear to me that in achieving those goals through plant-based nutrition, we also achieved a corollary result: we restored the body's own powerful capacity to resist and reverse vascular disease. Plant-based nutrition, it turns out, has a mighty beneficial effect on endothelial cells, those metabolic and biochemical dynamos that produce nitric oxide (see Figure 5). And nitric oxide, as I have noted, is absolutely essential

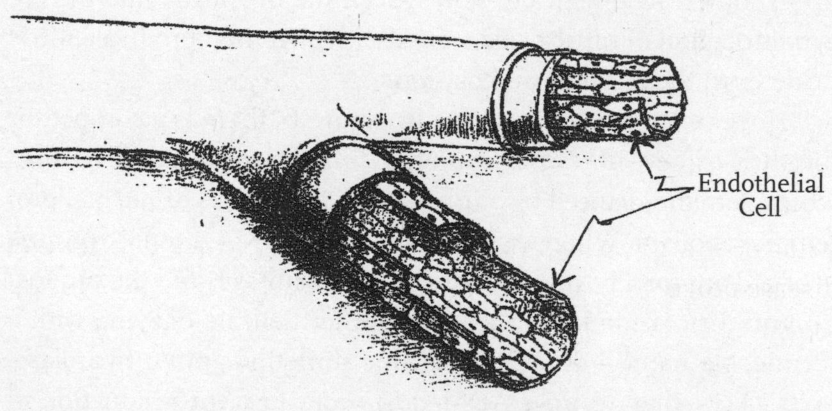

Figure 5. With plant-based nutrition, the endothelial cell is a metabolic dynamo that ensures vascular health.

to vascular health—a finding that won the Nobel Prize for Medicine in 1998.[8]

1. It relaxes blood vessels, selectively boosting blood flow to the organs that need it.

2. It prevents white blood cells and platelets from becoming sticky, and thus starting the buildup of vascular plaque.

3. It keeps the smooth muscle cells of arteries from growing into plaques.

4. It may even help to diminish vascular plaques once they are in place.

To understand how plant-based nutrition facilitates nitric oxide production, you need to have a sense of the biochemistry at play. The essential building block for nitric oxide production is a substance called L-arginine, an amino acid that is in rich supply in a variety of plant foods, especially legumes, beans, soy, and nuts. Figure 6 shows, schematically, how L-arginine fits neatly into the enzymatic action of nitric oxide synthase, which then produces nitric oxide from the arginine and oxygen.

However, as you can also see in Figure 6, there is a competitor for nitric oxide synthase: asymmetric dimethyl arginine, or ADMA, which is manufactured by our bodies in the course of normal protein metabolism. When we have too much ADMA, then L-arginine is edged out for a position in nitric oxide synthase, and the production of nitric oxide fails. There is another delicate enzyme with a formidable name—dimethyl arginine dimethyl amino hydrolase, or DDAH—that destroys ADMA, in order to favor production of nitric oxide. But the usual cardiovascular risk factors (high cholesterol, high triglycerides, high homocysteine, insulin resistance, hypertension, and tobacco use) all impair the ability of that delicate enzyme to destroy ADMA.

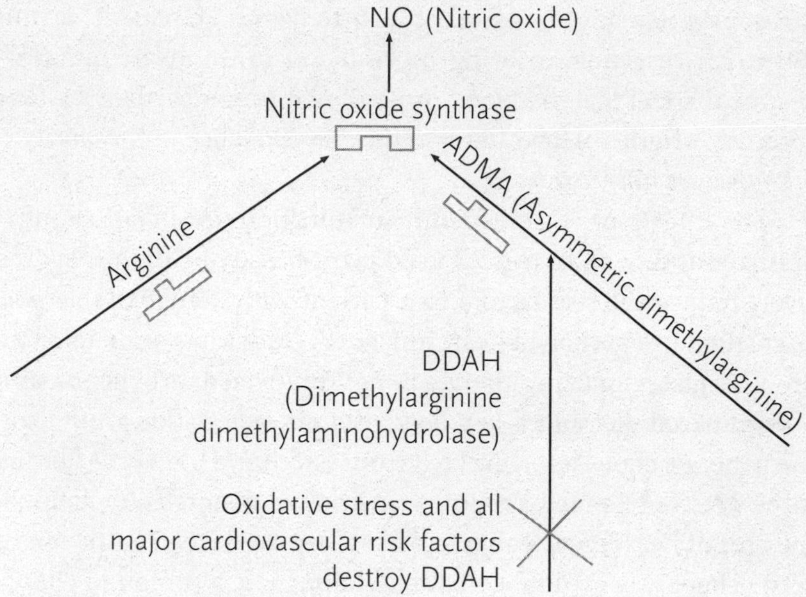

Figure 6. The pathway of nitric oxide production—arginine through nitric oxide synthase to nitric oxide—can be blocked by too much ADMA.

This biochemistry explains what is perhaps the key mechanism through which my patients became heart-attack–proof beyond twenty years. Their plant-based diet reduced or entirely eliminated all the above cardiovascular risk factors. The more compliant the patient, the more he or she reduced the risks.

Along the way, they also reduced symptoms such as angina pectoris—chest pain—perhaps the most frightening and incapacitating symptom of heart disease. Normally, physical effort or strong emotion causes the endothelium to go into action, producing nitric oxide, dilating the blood vessels, and thus boosting the flow of blood to the heart muscle. But in a patient with coronary disease, the endothelium's capacity is badly diminished. His narrowed coronary arteries do not dilate, and therefore his heart muscle does not receive the flow of blood it needs. The result: pain. It may be mild or it may be excruciating. Many patients become "cardiac cripples," terrified of exerting themselves physically, of making love, of expressing or experiencing strong emotions. To give such patients lasting relief, it is essential to bring more blood to the heart muscle—despite the fact that the blood must flow through partially blocked coronary arteries. How? *By restoring the endothelium's capacity to manufacture nitric oxide.*

The effects of a radical shift in nutrition are breathtaking—dramatic and swift. In 1996, I used plant-based nutrition to aggressively reduce the risk factors in a patient with demonstrably poor circulation to a portion of heart muscle. A cardiac pet scan noted the problem just prior to my intervention. Within ten days of her starting a plant-based diet and a low dose of a cholesterol-lowering drug, the patient's cholesterol level fell from 248 mg/dL to 137. After just three weeks of therapy, a repeat scan showed restored circulation to the area of heart muscle that had been deprived (see Figure 7 in insert). There was no doubt what had happened: a profound change in lifestyle, adopting strictly plant-based nutrition, brought about a rapid restoration of the endothelial cells' capacity to manufacture nitric oxide, and that, in turn, restored circulation.

That success led to a similar pilot study with Dr. Richard Brunken and Ray Go of the Cleveland Clinic Department of Nuclear Radiology and Dr. Kandice Marchant of the clinic's Department of Pathology. The results, shown in Figures 8, 9, 10, and 11 (see insert), confirm the ability of plant-based nutrition, in conjunction with cholesterol-reducing medication, to reperfuse—restore blood flow to—the heart muscle previously deprived of adequate circulation. I emphasize that this is not a case of the development of collaterals, naturally occurring bypasses, which take months or years to appear. The heart disease in these patients was long-standing, and the baseline study showed no reperfusion by collaterals; the reperfusion was observed three to twelve weeks after the patients made the lifestyle changes we outlined.

Students of physics will recognize this phenomenon as Poiseuille's Law, which describes the flow of liquid through hollow tubes. Think of a fire hose replacing a garden hose. Thus a modestly restored dilation of the blood vessels provides a huge increase in blood flow—clearly visible on the scans—and causes angina to disappear within weeks of starting therapy.

The endothelial system for enhancing and protecting our vascular system is brilliant. We can prevent it from breaking down, and we can restore it to good health even after a hazardous lifestyle has injured it. Just in case you are not yet convinced, let's take a look at what happened to the patients in my original study.

6

Living, Breathing Proof

DON FELTON'S WIFE, MACKIE, used to get up each morning and fry bacon, then make gravy from the grease, and serve it to Don over toast or homemade bread. "I loved it," Don says. "I ate it for years." And it wasn't just a matter of breakfast. "I remember side meat cooked in beans. Side meat was pure fat, a two-inch-thick piece of fat off the side of a pig, usually. The side meat is cured in salt, soaked overnight, rolled in cornmeal, and browned in a skillet with gravy made with the grease." Don Felton makes no bones about it: he *loved* gravy. And he loved a lot of other fatty foods, as well.

He arrived at my office on January 15, 1986. He was fifty-four, and had been informed by his cardiologist that—after twenty-seven years of chronic heart trouble and treatment, including a double bypass that had begun to fail—there was nothing more conventional medicine could do for him. As he walked across the skyway that connected my office with the rest of the Cleveland Clinic, he had to stop three or four times because of acute pain in his leg. An angiogram showed that the main artery in the leg was entirely blocked.

Don and Mackie talked with me for two hours about the program he was about to undertake. When they left my office, they stopped at a little Italian restaurant not far away and had a bowl of soup. "I guess this is the last good soup we will have," Don said to his wife. But he was, as he says, "at the end of the rope." He did not want to take a chance on more surgery. He was committed to my nutrition program, and began to follow it that very day.

After three or four months, Don Felton's chest pain eased. He no longer had to sleep propped up by pillows to ease the angina, which had been much worse when he lay down flat. And about seven months after he started the program, he mentioned that he had been so focused on his heart that he had forgotten to tell me about his leg: he now was able to walk across the skyway to my office without stopping—without a single stab of pain. I immediately sent him to the vascular laboratory for another pulse volume test, which showed that the flow of blood in the artery that had been blocked was back to normal (see Figure 12 in insert).

To me, Don is a test case in the power of the endothelial cells and how they respond to dramatically reduced cholesterol levels and lifestyle changes that eliminate all risk factors. And so, it turned out, were the rest of those who took part in my study. But anecdotal evidence of improved health is not sufficient to evaluate the results of this sort of research. I needed serious scientific information on just what was happening to participants in the study as they followed my program over the months and years.

Three separate measurements are necessary to evaluate results in this type of research:

1. Analysis of cholesterol levels during the course of the study.

2. Analysis of angiograms taken before, during, and after treatment.

3. Analysis of the clinical results of the study.

Keep in mind the background of the eighteen patients who stuck with the program. All had severe, progressive coronary heart disease.

In the eight years before my study began, all had received state-of-the-art cardiac care at the Cleveland Clinic. Collectively, they had experienced forty-nine cardiovascular events, including:

- Fifteen cases of increased angina
- Thirteen cases of measurable disease progression
- Seven cases of bypass surgery (in addition, two others in the group had had bypass surgery more than eight years before the study began)
- Four heart attacks
- Three strokes
- Two angioplasty procedures
- Two worsening stress tests

Here is how they fared in my study.

Cholesterol. During the first five years of the study, the patients' blood cholesterol was tested twice a month or more; for the next five years, it was tested once a month; and after that, every three months. The group began the study with an average blood cholesterol level of 246 mg/dL—a level all experts consider to be too high. By adhering to the nutrition program and using cholesterol-lowering drugs, they were able to reduce that group average to 137 mg/dL, cutting their cholesterol levels nearly in half. This is the most profound drop in cholesterol levels in such a study that I have been able to find in the medical literature, discounting recent studies using megadoses of statin.

Twelve years after joining the program, every one of the participants averaged total cholesterol below 150 mg/dL, the stated goal of the study. Their LDL—bad—cholesterol averaged 82 mg/dL, among the lowest ever reported in this type of study. Their good, HDL, cholesterol averaged 36.3 mg/dL, which is lower than the range generally accepted as normal. But it was sufficient to sustain the beneficial results. Our research strongly suggests, in fact, that lower than "normal" HDL levels are not worrisome as long as total cholesterol is well within the safe range—under 150 mg/dL—a finding that has been discussed by other researchers, as well.[1]

Angiograms. A coronary angiogram is a specialized X-ray of the coronary arteries. A flexible catheter is inserted into an artery, either at the elbow or the groin, and advanced toward the heart. At the entrance to the left ventricle, the heart's main pumping chamber, the catheter can be alternately inserted into each of the coronary arteries. Dye is injected through the catheter into each coronary artery while a running film (cine-angiogram) captures a precise picture of the artery and its major branches.

When these angiogram pictures are taken over time, it is possible to compare them and thus to measure how diseased portions of the arteries are faring. Are they remaining the same? Are they getting worse—narrowing as they sustain further blockage? Or are they improving—growing wider, and thus allowing more oxygen and nutrients to reach the heart muscle? These analyses of the films must be scrupulously precise and objective. For my study, all were performed three times. In addition, to avoid any possibility of bias, the technicians who performed the angiogram analyses were "blinded"—that is, they did not know whether the film they were analyzing was the initial, baseline film taken before the patient joined the study, or the follow-up film taken upon its completion.

At the five-year mark, seven of the eighteen participants were unable to have a follow-up angiogram. The results I report here are for the eleven participants who did have follow-up angiograms after five years. The analyses were stunning. In sustaining cholesterol readings below 150 mg/dL, these patients eliminated any clinical progression of their disease. Every single one arrested progression of the heart disease, and eight participants actually selectively reversed it. Some of the reversals were striking, as you can see in the photographs that accompany this text. Figure 13 (see insert) shows a 10 percent reversal of disease over five years in the left anterior descending coronary artery of a sixty-seven-year-old pediatrician. Figure 14 shows a 20 percent improvement in the circumflex coronary artery of a fifty-eight-year-old factory worker. Figure 15 shows a 30 percent improvement in the right coronary artery of a fifty-four-year-old security guard. Again, see the agiogram of Dr. Joe Crowe, revealing total disease reversal after thirty-two months (Figure 1).

Having angiographic proof of disease reversal was an occasion of enormous joy for study participants and cause for family gatherings and champagne toasts. It was also enormously gratifying for me. It showed, beyond argument, that the hypothesis and foundation of the research was solid. We now had irrefutable scientific evidence that heart disease could be arrested and reversed. And if it can be reversed it can also be prevented.

Clinical results. Before discussing the clinical results, it is important to review the one death that occurred during the study. The patient was a man in his sixties who had severe coronary artery disease. He had been accepted into the study two weeks after sustaining a massive heart attack during an unsuccessful angioplasty. His unstable condition persisted and seven months later he underwent bypass surgery. His left heart chamber was so badly damaged and scarred that it was able to pump blood at less than 20 percent of its normal capacity.

Such patients have a very poor outlook. Nevertheless, this man survived. And after he had spent nearly five years on the program, a follow-up angiogram compared four of the areas where his arteries had narrowed. Two were unchanged. Two had improved.

Ten months later, he died of a cardiac arrhythmia. Postmortem study showed no new blockages or heart attacks. Despite the improving coronary artery blood supply and decrease in angina, his heart, which was so scarred, had literally electrocuted itself into arrest.

As for the rest of the group, all improved. Nine of the patients had come to the study with angina—pain in the heart muscle caused by inadequate blood supply. It was completely eliminated in two and much improved in the remaining seven, including the patient who died. Exercise capacity improved. Sexual activity was enhanced. One patient confided that the impotence that had long bothered him had been cured in the course of the study.

The results have lasted over the years. Don Felton, who could barely manage the walk to my office when he first came to see me, is now in his seventies—fit and active. "When I first started, I was down," he says. "Now, I've been eating this way for so long I don't think about it anymore." Mackie still makes him gravy, but she makes it with fat-free broth, and he pours it over mashed potatoes. And Don still goes deer-hunting every year. But there are a few differences from the old days. For one, he takes oatmeal on the trips so he doesn't miss his healthy breakfasts. For another, he doesn't eat venison anymore.

Emil Huffgard, once such a prisoner of nitroglycerin, unable even to sleep unless he was in a sitting position, improved quickly after starting to eat right and to reduce his cholesterol. He had worked for the telephone company as an engineer, but had been forced to retire early because of his health. About six months after he joined the study, he came to my office and, with tears in his eyes, said, "If I continue to improve this much, I'll have to go back to work!" And despite his wife's worry that he might not make it to their daughter's wedding, he was able to walk her down the aisle after all. Eleven years after Emil joined the program, an angiogram confirmed that he had achieved some reversal of his disease.

(Don and Emil, both of whom had undergone bypass surgery before joining the study, teach an important lesson in the downside of that procedure: the vessels used for bypassing blocked arteries simply cannot last forever. Eventually, they scar shut. In Don's case, a vein had been used to bypass his clogged coronary artery. It lasted for twenty years—about twice as long as most vein bypasses—but eventually had to be replaced. In Emil's case, an artery had been used for the bypass, and it lasted for fully thirty years. At the end of that time, it suddenly blocked, causing a mild heart attack and requiring a corrective bypass. In both men, the reversal of disease in their native coronary arteries, due to their compliance during the course of our study, enabled them to tolerate the required surgery safely. Today, both are well, free of angina or any restriction on their activity.)

Jerry Murphy, the company executive whose male family members had all died young as far back as anyone could remember, is, as I write, in his mid-eighties. During fourteen years on our program, he maintained a total cholesterol level below 120 mg/dL. The patient who was once called "a heart attack about to happen" by his cardiologist jogged every day until he was seventy-eight. Today, he is beginning to experience a bit of arthritis—something no other male members of his family ever had. None lived long enough to acquire it.

Evelyn Oswick, whose doctor had told her to go home, find a rocker, and wait to die, is now in her late seventies. Despite her initial skepticism, once she made up her mind about my nutrition program, she never turned back. And her heart disease, as a result, is completely under control. In fact today, when Evelyn sees a new doctor, she tells him she no longer has heart disease. With characteristic self-confidence, she declares that anyone who has a heart attack these days is simply foolish, since there's such solid information on how to arrest the disease.

Jim Trusso, who had so much trouble with the program when he joined the group, stayed with it. His wife, Sue, says that even today, he "is not a fruit-and-vegetable person." But he knew that changing his eating habits was the only way he could save himself. And little by little, he learned to live with the diet, how to season healthy foods so that he grew to enjoy them. Shortly after I wrote the twelve-year follow-up report on my patients, Jim joined a charity event, bicycling from Cleveland to Toledo and back—a round-trip of approximately 225 miles. He was definitely overdoing the exercise, and sustained a cardiac arrest during the exertion. (This was not a heart attack, but rather a case of building up epinephrine through exercise and then stopping suddenly; with his muscles no longer consuming the epinephrine, it caused arrhythmia and Jim's heart stopped beating.) He was resuscitated, and an angiogram suggested that he needed a third bypass to more fully protect him in his active lifestyle. His strong constitution withstood the surgery.

Now in his sixties, Jim has retired from the education system—he ultimately became superintendent of schools—but he is hardly sitting still. He bikes on the beach every day, between eight and ten miles. He kayaks, lectures at the local arboretum, and travels the world with Sue. And to this day, he maintains his cholesterol level at 121 mg/dL. He won the bet with the doctor who wagered a steak dinner than he would never get his cholesterol level below 305. But he has never collected—for obvious reasons!

Jack Robinson also made a bet with his cardiologist. Two years after he refused bypass surgery and started my nutrition plan, his doctor in Akron was still deeply concerned about Jack's choice. He suggested the following wager: Jack would have another angiogram, and if it showed further progression of disease, he would agree to have the bypass. The angiogram did not show disease progression. Quite the contrary, it showed that Jack was *reversing* the effects of his disease.

Ultimately, Jack moved to Piqua, Ohio, where he signed on with a new cardiologist. Like Jack's old doctor, the new one was skeptical of Jack's nutrition-based approach, and in 1998, Jack reluctantly agreed to have yet another angiogram. This one revealed even further improvement—so much, in fact, that to Jack's dismay, the cardiologist began boasting that it was his drug regime that had made all the difference.

What has occurred with all these people is very basic: the blood supply through their coronary arteries to their heart muscle has improved. In the majority of patients, the arteries themselves are measurably wider. Profound reduction of cholesterol has increased the capacity of the endothelium, the arteries' inner lining, to produce nitric oxide, which in turn dilates the arteries themselves—even diseased arteries. And that's not the only improvement. Recent research indicates that reducing blood cholesterol levels decreases the thickness of the membrane surrounding red blood cells, thus enhancing its permeability. This allows the red cells to pick up oxygen more readily as they pass through the lungs, and enables them to release the oxygen more efficiently as they circulate through the heart muscle. Finally, the patients' plant-based diet, eliminating the ingestion of foods that injure vascular tissues, has restored strength and integrity to the endothelium as a whole. Any plaques in these patients were protectively capped and could not rupture or initiate the cascade of clotting that defines a heart attack (see Figure 16 in insert).

These patients are now heart-attack–proof.

Three of the original members of the study have died since it ended. One died of pulmonary fibrosis. The second vomited violently, collapsed, and died amid copious bleeding about thirteen years after he entered the program. No autopsy was ever performed, but because of the vomiting and bleeding, which are not associated with heart disease, I suspect he died of Mallory-Weiss syndrome, in which a gastric artery is eroded by acid and retching. The third was a retired truck driver, who fell into a terrible depression. At the time of his death, he was living in a facility where he couldn't eat safely, and little by little, his health deteriorated.

In 1998, I reviewed the status of the six patients who were released from the study in the first twelve to fifteen months, and returned to their cardiologists and prestudy diet. In every one of them, the heart disease had grown worse. All told, since leaving the study, they had suffered:

- Four cases of increased angina
- Two episodes of ventricular tachycardia (a potentially lethal arrhythmia, or disruption of the heartbeat, which causes the heart to race)
- Four bypass operations
- One angioplasty

- One case of congestive heart failure

- One death from complications of arrhythmia

What a contrast! As I have reported, the patients who stayed with the program collectively had sustained no fewer than forty-nine cardiac events in the years leading up to the study. One man, six years into the program, went back to his old eating habits during an eighteen-month period of hectic business activity, and his angina, which had disappeared, returned, requiring bypass surgery. That was the only case of a new cardiac event among participants in the study during the first twelve years. There was another case of bypass surgery that I learned about while writing this book, but I do not count it as a true coronary event. The patient in question left the Cleveland area two years after joining the study, and I lost contact with him. He continued to follow the nutrition program—and does even now, twenty years later—but he told me that he insisted upon the bypass surgery in order to hasten relief from symptoms that kept him from improving his tennis.

Among the fully compliant patients, during the twelve-year study, there was not one further clinical episode of worsening coronary artery disease after they committed themselves to keeping cholesterol within the safe range.

All of these patients have continued, on their own, to follow the nutritional program and cholesterol-lowering medication I recommended, even though the study has ended. As they reflect upon nearly two decades of freedom from disease, these patients are empowered by the knowledge that they have taken control of their own health, and have taken into their own hands the treatment of the disease that was destroying their lives.

Anthony Yen, whose New Year's weekend in 1987 nearly turned into a deadly debacle, puts it perfectly. One of his five bypasses had failed just before he joined the study, and he was determined to keep the disease from growing worse. He remembers how tough it was to follow the program at first, having to keep the detailed diary of what he consumed, and facing blood tests every two weeks.

But suddenly, one day a month or so into the program, Anthony realized he felt dramatically better. "I walked in the wind, and had no angina," he says. He turned to his wife, Joseanne, and spoke triumphant words any one of the study participants would endorse: "We won the battle!"

7

Why Didn't Anyone Tell Me?

ONE OF THE LONGTIME FOLLOWERS of my nutrition plan is a man named Abraham Brickner, now retired, who was the Cleveland Clinic's director of health services, research and program development. Abe's mother died of heart disease when she was sixty-two. His brother had bypass surgery at the age of fifty-five and died from his heart disease a decade later. One of Abe's nephews had a heart attack at forty-five; a second nephew died from a heart attack at forty-two. Abe had his first bypass at fifty-five, and his second at sixty-five.

Although he began to modify his eating habits somewhat after the first surgery, for most of his life, Abe had eaten a high-fat diet: aged steaks from his father's grocery fried in butter; freshers—half a pound of corned beef on a heel of bread; chopped liver with schmaltz, which is pure chicken fat, once a week; a big plate of waffles after the movies on Saturday nights. Abe, a career health-care planner and consumer advocate, had paid considerable attention to health matters over the years. And as he says: "When a cholesterol of 250 was normal, I met the standard."

When a cholesterol of 250 was normal. It is hard to believe, but for decades, it was the conventional wisdom that blood levels of cholesterol up to 300 mg/dL were perfectly normal. Over the years, the advice from the "experts" has varied, and consumers of health care have been understandably confused about what cholesterol level should be their goal. It has been a constantly moving target. Most recently, national health organizations—the American Heart Association, the National Cholesterol Education Program, and the National Research Council—have decreed that serum cholesterol should be below 200 mg/dL.[1] These same organizations suggest limiting fat consumption to no more than 30 percent of the calories consumed each day.

But that level of fat consumption has never been shown to arrest or reverse coronary artery disease. Quite the contrary, research has shown that while cutting fat consumption to that level from even higher levels may help to slow the disease's progression, the disease, nonetheless, will progress.

The truth is that the medical profession knows better. We have known for a long time that one out of every four persons who have heart attacks has a blood cholesterol level between 180 and 210 mg/dL,[2] and we know that more than a third of those in the Framingham Heart Study who had heart disease showed cholesterol levels between 150 and 200 mg/dL.[3] That means that millions of Americans who are doing the best they can to meet the standards set by national health officials are, in spite of their efforts, getting sick.

Here's a clear, plain English translation of what our government and the national health agencies have done: they have chosen a "safe" cholesterol level for the public that virtually guarantees—if everyone actually met their stated goal—that every year more than 1.2 million Americans will suffer heart attacks and that millions more will watch the inevitable progression of their coronary artery disease.

What is going on here? If the evidence is so clear that the goal for cholesterol levels should be set below 150 mg/dL, why don't the national experts and policy makers tell us that? When we ask representatives of our government to establish safe levels of bacteria in our drinking water, they do not select a level at which a substantial proportion of the population will contract cholera and dysentery;

instead, they set a level that guarantees none of us will be infected. The case is similar with official standards for other contaminants. We do not choose a level at which 20 percent of our children will develop lead-induced brain disease from lead in the water. We choose a level that ensures the safety of everyone. So why is the policy so different when it comes to levels of cholesterol in the blood?

The answer lies in a complex blend of culture, habit, taste, realpolitik, and other factors—including, frankly, a somewhat condescending attitude among medical experts toward the lay public. Let's look at the facts.

To begin with, it is true that people have a craving for oil, dairy, and animal fat, and that includes the medical scientists who study the problem. We are immersed in an environment of toxic food that is attractive, tasteful, reasonably priced, and heavily advertised. And there are powerful commercial interests that want no change in the American diet. Over the years, there have been a number of attempts to bring nutritional recommendations more into line with what the science actually shows. In every case, intensive lobbying by industry—the producers and purveyors of dairy products, meat, and poultry—has caused those who set the standards to pull their punches.

To put it quite simply, the fox is in the henhouse. Nowhere is this more apparent than at the United States Department of Agriculture, which since the late 1970s has been issuing the government's official guidelines on what American citizens should be eating. In a recent editorial for *Nutrition Action Health Letter,* a publication of the Center for Science in the Public Interest, Michael Jacobsen named the major officeholders in the USDA and described what each had done for a living before going to work for the Department of Agriculture.[4] Every single one had previously been employed by the dairy, meat, or poultry industry. And as recently as October 2000, the Physicians Committee for Responsible Medicine successfully litigated to find out exactly who was compensating the members of the USDA's U.S. Dietary Guidelines Committee. It turned out that six of the eleven committee members, including the chairman, had financial ties to the food industry.

In my opinion, the Department of Agriculture, which by definition is supposed to protect and promote the nation's agricultural interests, should disqualify itself from responsibility for setting nutrition standards. That duty belongs more properly to the Centers for Disease Control and Prevention. But so far, the USDA still holds the power to advise Americans on what they should be eating, and every five years, when it updates its advice, its guidelines end up misleading the public and betraying the science. As long ago as 1991, for example, proposed changes in the food pyramid would have relegated meat and dairy foods to lesser importance. But by the time the lobbying was finished, the USDA agreed on a misleading compromise for the new proposals that still emphasized consumption of animal protein.

Not much has changed since then. Here are some examples, drawn from a written critique I delivered to the 2005 Food Guidelines Committee:

1. USDA Recommendation: "Consume three or more ounce-equivalents of whole-grain products per day, with the rest of the recommended grains coming from whole-grain products. In general, at least half the grains should come from whole grains."

   In other words, the other half of the grains consumed may come from refined grains, which have lost many of their natural nutrients and fiber content—and which cause elevated levels of triglycerides in the bloodstream, a recognized risk factor in coronary artery disease.

2. USDA Recommendation: "Consume three cups per day of fat-free or low-fat milk or equivalent milk products."

   Even low-fat milk contains significant amounts of saturated fat, which will clog arteries. In addition, fully 50 million Americans are lactose intolerant. For them, ingesting milk causes gastrointestinal upsets. Milk consumption has also been linked to the development of prostate cancer. Casein, the major protein in milk, has been shown in animal studies to powerfully promote cancer growth.[5]

3. USDA recommendation: "Consume less than 10 percent of calories from saturated fat and less than 300 mg/day of cholesterol, and keep *trans*-fatty acid consumption as low as possible."

   This is strange, impractical advice. I don't know of any food scientist, nutritionist, physician, or other expert who, on a daily basis, would go to the enormous trouble of calculating how many calories' worth of saturated fat they are ingesting, or who have more than a general notion of how many milligrams of cholesterol and trans fat they consume. It is absurd to ask the public to follow rules that even the scientists who invent them do not. It would be far simpler—and clearer—to advise people to avoid animal-based products (the source of all cholesterol and most saturated fat) and also to avoid products labeled "hydrogenated" or "partially hydrogenated," since these contain the most harmful trans fats.

4. USDA recommendation: "Keep total fat intake between 20 to 35 percent of calories, with most fats coming from sources of polyunsaturated and monounsaturated fat, such as fish, nuts, and vegetable oils."

   This recommendation is of major concern. In effect, your government is suggesting a level of fat consumption that cannot arrest vascular disease and—quite the contrary—has actually been shown to promote it. In Chapter 10, I will discuss the documented harmful effects of monounsaturated oils. But fish consumption poses a set of dangers all its own. Filled with toxins such as PCBs and mercury, fish are a known hazard—so much so that pregnant women are advised to cat them sparingly. And the development of fish farming, made necessary by the steady depletion of the Earth's oceans, poses some new dangers. Fish farming is so unhealthy that its products must be treated with antibiotics, and many health authorities advise against eating farm-grown fish. There is no doubt that the omega-3 fatty acids found in fish are valuable, but there are other, safer sources of these acids, which I will discuss in Chapter 8.

5. USDA recommendation: "When selecting and preparing meat, poultry, dry beans, and milk or milk products, make choices that are lean, low-fat, or fat-free."

   This is largely obfuscation—confusing and misleading for the vast majority of people who are unfamiliar with the science. There are no fat-free meats. Some meat is merely less fat than other meat—and thus slightly less toxic. The same is true of poultry. And that's just the start of the problem. Mass-produced poultry is so contaminated with bacteria that poultry inspectors, intimately acquainted with its condition, rarely consume it. In fact, you are regularly advised by our health experts not to allow it to infect foods in your refrigerator or on your countertop. As for milk and milk products, they have been clearly implicated in the development of heart disease, strokes, hypertension, diabetes, osteoporosis, and prostate cancer. And their labeling can be very misleading indeed. Are you under the impression that milk labeled "2%" delivers only 2 percent of its calories from fat (as compared with whole milk, which delivers 55 percent of its calories from fat)? Wrong. In fact, 35 percent of the calories from "2%" milk are from fat. Similarly, 21 percent of the calories in "1%" milk are from fat.

How can it be that an arm of the United States government would design and promote dietary guidelines that, if followed, guarantee that millions of Americans will perish prematurely? This is an international embarrassment and a public health disaster. The truth is that giving the U.S. Department of Agriculture, as presently configured, the responsibility for issuing such guidelines is much like inviting Al Capone to prepare your income tax returns.

But our medical organizations have also waffled when it comes to this subject. Although they have been advising us for well over a decade that dairy products, oil, and animal fat are bad for us, and although it becomes clearer with every passing year that vascular disease, cancer, and other illnesses are the direct result of the toxic Western diet, these organizations just cannot bring themselves to radically change nutritional recommendations. Instead, the experts keep suggesting that we reduce consumption of animal and dairy fats, that we eat red meat only once or twice a week, for example, and that we remove the skin from chicken—advice that is imprecise and vague and does not significantly reduce fat intake.

Almost all experts will agree that coronary artery disease is rarely seen in individuals with cholesterol levels consistently below 150 mg/dL. Almost all would also agree that reducing fat intake to less than 10 percent of calories consumed will help mightily in achieving low cholesterol levels. And they would concede that it is impossible to eat a diet built around meat, poultry, dairy products, and oil, and still derive less than 10 percent of calories from fat.

But rather than state these facts clearly to the public, rather than set a truly safe level of blood cholesterol and advise Americans how they can achieve it, the experts balk—often explaining that the public might have an overwhelming sense of frustration at not being able to comply with the nutrition changes necessary.

I think this is wrong. We should tell the public what is healthiest for them. People will decide for themselves whether they wish to comply. We, as scientists, must at least tell them what is optimal.

In 1991, I assembled a blue-ribbon faculty nationally known and respected for their expertise in cardiology, nutrition, pathology, pediatrics, epidemiology, and public health for the First National Conference on Lipids in the Elimination and Prevention of Coronary Artery Disease. During two days of presentations in Tucson, Arizona, these scientists were challenged to develop what they felt constituted the optimal diet for health, one least likely to develop coronary artery disease. I asked them to answer the question: What do you tell the patient who says, "I'll do anything, but I never want to have heart disease," or, "I have had a heart attack, and I never want another"?

One panelist replied, "Have him eat beans, beans, and more beans." Another, Professor T. Colin Campbell of Cornell, one of the world's most respected nutritionists and coauthor of *The China Study,* said most clearly and forcibly what other faculty members were feeling:

"If we are reasonably sure of what our data from these studies are telling us, then why must we be reticent about recommending a diet which we know is safe and healthy? Scientists can no longer take the attitude that the public cannot benefit from information they are not ready for. We must have the integrity to tell them the truth and let them decide what to do with it. We cannot force them to follow the guidelines we recommend, but we can give them these guidelines and then let them decide. I personally have great faith in the public. We must tell them that a diet of roots, stems, seeds, flowers, fruit, and leaves is the healthiest diet and the only diet we can promote, endorse, and recommend."[6]

Following the conference, I prepared a summary that was ultimately approved by ten of the thirteen faculty participants. The following four paragraphs reveal the strong stand of these acknowledged experts—and might serve as a model for more useful nutritional advice for Americans than what the U.S. government and national health organizations currently provide:

"Present governmental and national heath organization guidelines do not provide a maximal opportunity to either arrest or prevent coronary artery disease. Studies demonstrate persons following present guidelines will have increased rates of disease progression when compared to persons achieving lower serum lipid levels through diet and/or lipid-lowering drugs.

"A diet which would achieve superior results in reducing atherosclerosis would be a 10–15 percent fat diet provided largely by grains, legumes, vegetables, and fruit. This diet offers protection against the common neoplasms of breast, prostate, colon, and ovary. It also lessens the likelihood of developing obesity, hypertension, strokes, and adult-onset diabetes. There are no known adverse effects of such a diet when mineral and vitamin contents are adequate.

"Children and adolescents require major attention to develop early habits of optimal nutrition. Schools should assume a significant leadership role in achieving this goal.

"Speculation about the degree of public compliance must not influence the accuracy of the recommendations."[7]

Indisputably, in recommending that Americans convert to plant-based nutrition, we would be asking Americans to undertake profound taste transitions. But there are some potential allies in the cause: the professional chefs of the world, those employed by upscale hotels, restaurants, businesses, clubs, and other venues that require food of exquisite taste, texture, variety, and presentation. These chefs are masters at achieving delightful meals no matter what the basic foods.

Several years ago, I was invited to speak about arresting and reversing heart disease at a luncheon meeting of health maintenance organization directors at the Broadmoor Hotel in Colorado Springs. I agreed to speak on one condition: if I could be responsible for the luncheon menu. The planners of the HMO convention agreed.

After my presentation, one doubting audience member declared that nobody would eat a diet consisting of 10 percent fat or less.

"Did you enjoy your lunch?" I asked.

"Yes, it was delicious," he replied.

"Fine," I answered. "You should know that it was 10 percent fat, which was my requirement of the chef if I were to speak here today."

Point made, with the help of a master chef. Unfortunately, he may have been an exception. A decade ago, I was asked to make a presentation for a highly respected culinary institute. By the time I arrived, the director had decided that he did not want his chefs-in-training to hear what I had to say, since it clearly conflicted with what they were being taught; instead, I gave a thumbnail sketch of my data to a much smaller audience—the director and his assistant. A few years later, I was asked to speak at another meeting, the annual national chefs' convention in Nashville, Tennessee. I presided at a special breakout session with approximately twenty chefs, all of whom had coronary artery disease. They'd been done in by their own cooking.

The good news is that the word is spreading. Americans are steadily growing more health conscious. Since I started my research twenty years ago, there has been a marked increase in the number of experts who believe that nutrition plays a critical role in helping you maintain safe cholesterol levels and in protecting you from the common killer diseases, especially from coronary artery disease.

And many laymen come to that understanding on their own. A few years after his first bypass surgery, Abe Brickner joined a study of people who had undergone the operation. "I began to sense from my reading that something was going on," he says. "If 50 percent of people go back for a second bypass, I wanted to know what was in store for me." Through the study, Abe had another angiogram, which led to his second bypass surgery when he was sixty-five. But as he says today, "If I had the knowledge base I have now, I would not even have had the first bypass." That second surgery provided "the final flash of insight and self-awareness, and sent me into the preventive mode. I was ready when Dr. Esselstyn came along."

It took hand-holding to get Abe past his cravings for the fat-filled diet he had enjoyed for so many years. But he committed himself to my nutrition plan, and he has stuck with it ever since. His cholesterol dropped from 235 mg/dL to 123, where it remains to this day. Now in his eighties, Abe Brickner is convinced that he will live to be one hundred. Best of all, he says, "The locus of control is *me*! The doctor isn't responsible for my health—I am."

8

Simple Steps

YOU, TOO, can take control of your heart disease. This chapter—perhaps the most important in this book for those who have heart disease or people who simply never want to develop it—will tell you exactly how to go about it.

As you already have learned, my approach to this potentially lethal disease is vigorous and sustained. The technique I recommend is based entirely on my research and supported by twelve years of formal study and twenty years of continuing work with a diverse group of patients. And its success depends very much on acute attention to detail. In the words of Rupert Turnbull, a former surgeon at the Cleveland Clinic: "Inappropriate application of the method is no excuse for its abandonment!"

Here, once again, is the basic message of my research: no one who achieves and maintains total blood cholesterol of 150 mg/dL and LDL levels below 80 mg/dL—using strict plant-based nutrition and, where necessary, low doses of cholesterol-reducing drugs—experiences progression of heart disease. Many, in fact, are able to rejoice at clear medical evidence that they have actually *reversed* the effects of their disease.

Recall that three-quarters of the population of this planet has never known heart disease. Your cholesterol metabolism and, with it, your resistance to the insidious progression of heart disease, can come to resemble those of the rural Chinese, the residents of Okinawa, the Tarahumara Indians of Northern Mexico, the Papua Highlanders of New Guinea, and many native Africans. Among these peoples, because of the plant-based diets they have always consumed, heart disease is virtually unknown. I am convinced from my research and from counseling hundreds of patients with heart disease that you, like them, can make yourself heart-attack–proof.

In my initial interviews with all potential patients, I stress the need for total commitment. My first request is that patients and their families eliminate from their vocabulary, from their thinking, from their most basic belief systems, the phrase "This little bit can't hurt." If you have retained only one fact from my explanations of the science behind this program, I hope it is this: that just a little bit of forbidden food—fats, dairy products, oils, animal proteins—*can* hurt, and will. Think of it this way: if you adopt a healthy diet overall, but allow yourself to have fats just two or three times a week, that means you are abusing and injuring yourself on one hundred fifty or so days of the year. This "moderation" rationale will deprive you of the ultimate health benefits of plant-based nutrition. Just "this little bit" is enough to prevent you from remaining free of heart disease.

If you understand and accept that premise, you are 95 percent of the way toward success in arresting your disease. Occasional exceptions, however modest, undermine results. (I must confess: on every New Year's Eve, I consume eight to ten chocolate peanut butter cups.)

I am reminded of a breakfast several years ago when I was invited to speak at a conference on breast cancer. Joining me at the meal was a distinguished East Coast surgeon who was also participating in the conference. Eighteen months earlier, he had had a heart attack. Even so, he was eating pancakes dripping with butter and a side order of bacon. Seeing my raised eyebrows, the surgeon explained that he ordinarily ate carefully, and allowed himself to go off his diet only on weekends, when out of town, or on special occasions.

Since then, he has sustained a massive stroke, which deprived him of normal speech. The same vascular disease that narrows the coronary arteries to the heart narrows the arteries to the brain.

With the understanding that total commitment is the order of the day, let's proceed to the rules of my nutrition plan.

First, the foods to avoid:

1. **Anything with a face or a mother.** This includes meat, poultry, fish, and eggs. You may be aware that arginine and omega-3 fatty acids, which are essential to endothelial health and other bodily functions, are plentiful in fish. But there are other, healthier sources of these substances, which I will discuss when I recommend dietary supplements for those on my program.

2. **Dairy products.** That means butter, cheese, cream, ice cream, yogurt, and milk—even skim milk.

3. **Oils.** *All* oils, including virgin olive oil and canola oil. (For more on this subject, please see Chapter 10.)

4. **Refined grains.** These, unlike whole grains, have been stripped of much of their fiber and nutrients. You should avoid white rice and "enriched" flour products, which are found in many pastas, breads, bagels, and baked goods.

5. **Nuts.** Those who have heart disease should avoid all nuts. Those without disease can consume walnuts in moderation because they can provide considerable omega-3 fatty acids, which are important for many essential bodily functions. But I am extremely wary of nuts. Although

short-term studies funded by nut companies show that they may positively affect good and bad cholesterol, I know of no long-term studies indicating that they can arrest and reverse heart disease, and patients may easily overingest them, elevating their cholesterol levels.

Now, for the foods you are allowed—in fact, encouraged—to consume. This list, although it may not include many of the products you used to eat, permits you to fill your plate with a delicious and colorful array of foods brimming with fiber, nutrients, and antioxidants, all essential to heart health and overall well-being:

1. **Vegetables.** This is by no means a complete list, but it gives you a good sense of the wide variety of vegetables that you can eat. Sweet potatoes, yams, potatoes (but never French fried or prepared in any other way that involves adding fats!). Broccoli, kale, and spinach. Asparagus, artichokes, eggplant, radishes, celery, onions, carrots. Brussels sprouts, corn, cabbages, lettuces, peppers. Bok choy, Swiss chard, and beet greens. Turnips and parsnips. Summer squashes, winter squashes, tomatoes (although strictly speaking, tomatoes are fruit), cucumbers. Almost any vegetable you can imagine is legal on this plan, with a single exception, for cardiac patients: avocados, which carry a high fat content unusual for vegetables. Those without heart disease can eat avocados as long as their blood lipid levels are not elevated.

2. **Legumes.** Beans, peas, and lentils of all kinds. This is a wide-ranging family of plants, and you are almost certain to discover delicious varieties you may never have encountered before embarking on this nutrition plan.

3. **Whole grains.** Whole wheat, whole rye, bulgur wheat, whole oats, barley, buckwheat (kasha or buckwheat groats),

whole corn, cornmeal, wild rice, brown rice, popcorn, and less well-known whole grains, such as couscous, kamut (a relative of durum wheat), quinoa, amaranth, millet, spelt, teff, triticale, grano, and faro. There is a marvelous variety of choices, both familiar and new. You can also eat cereals that do not contain added sugar and oil—old-fashioned oats, for instance (not the quick-cooking variety), shredded wheat, and brand names like Grape-Nuts. Breads should be whole grain, and should not contain added oil. Whole-grain pastas are allowed—those made from whole wheat, brown rice, spelt, and quinoa. (Be careful about restaurant pasta. It is often egg-based and made from white flour, and there may well be oil lurking in the marinara sauce.)

4. **Fruit.** Fruits of all varieties are permitted. A word of caution is in order, however: it is preferable to limit your fruit consumption to three pieces a day (or, for berries and grapes, three servings, each about the size of a modest handful). It is also best to avoid drinking pure fruit juices. Fruit—and juice, especially—carries a high sugar content, and consuming too much of it rapidly raises the blood sugar. The body compensates to the sugar high with a surge of insulin from the pancreas—and the insulin, in turn, stimulates the liver to manufacture more cholesterol.[1] It may also elevate triglyceride levels. Be careful of sugar-laden desserts, which can have the same effect.

5. **Beverages.** Water, seltzer water (try adding a small amount of fruit juice to boost flavor), oat milk, no-fat soy milk, coffee, and tea. And alcohol is just fine, in moderation. (That's something my colleague and patient Joe Crowe appreciates. There's an annual Robert Burns party that celebrates the poet and other things Scottish, and its centerpiece is a feast—featuring, among other things,

haggis, which is made of the lungs, heart, and other suet-laden innards of a sheep or calf. There's only one thing on the menu, Joe points out, that someone on my nutrition plan can consume: the Scotch whisky!)

Ideally, most of the food you buy for this nutrition plan—much of it fresh produce—will not require labels. But for products that do, be sure you study the ingredients very carefully.

Here's why. In recent years, the U.S. Food and Drug Administration has forced the food industry to label fat content of foods more accurately than it did in the past. However, there is at least one very important loophole in the labeling rules. The FDA allows manufacturers to say that a product contains zero fat per serving if one serving contains 1/2 gram of fat or less. So imagine a box of doughnuts, each of which contains 1 gram of fat. Under the new system, the manufacturers simply state on the box that the six doughnuts inside represent twelve servings—i.e., that a single serving equals half a doughnut. Since half a doughnut would contain just 1/2 gram of fat, they can legally declare that the doughnuts contain zero fat per serving.

That, of course, is nonsense. These "no fat" products may contain less fat overall than their higher octane counterparts, but hidden in "no fat" salad dressings, cheeses, breakfast pastries, and spreads is the same old dairy, animal, and oil fat, and it will destroy your health. Be on the lookout for phrases like "contains negligible amounts of fat." Scrutinize lists of ingredients for any mention of oil, of monoglycerides and diglycerides, of hydrogenated or partially hydrogenated oils or glycerin. Remember, a pig with lipstick and earrings is still a pig. A year of consuming these "zero fat" products will actually add pounds of lethal fat to your diet.

Jim Trusso, one of the patients in my study, learned the hard way. For six careful years on the program, he never touched meat, dairy products, or oils. But suddenly, his cholesterol spiked over 200 mg/dL. It didn't take us long to figure out what the problem was. Jim had not been much of a fan of fruits and vegetables before joining the study, and in those first years on the program, he was always looking for ways to avoid them. When the no-fat products began appearing on supermarket shelves, he was thrilled—and happily added them to his diet. He reformed quickly after the cholesterol scare, and has been back in control ever since, maintaining a total cholesterol of 120 mg/dL.

Truly no-fat products are increasingly available—including some salad dressings, crackers, chips, pretzels, and cookies. Look carefully. Scrutinize labels. Pay attention to the lists of ingredients. And when in doubt, don't be shy about calling the manufacturers. A talk with a company's chief dietitian or medical consultant will give you a straight answer on fat content.

So now, you've committed yourself to eating only the legal foods listed above, and to avoiding all of the categories I do not allow. Is there anything else you need to consume to make sure you're on the right course for optimal heart health?

Consuming the full range of plant-based nutrition does not require supplemental calcium or a multivitamin. However, for all those who are consuming plant-based nutrition, I recommend the following supplements:

1. **Vitamin B_{12}**. I favor 1000 mcg (micrograms) daily.

2. **Vitamin D_3**. Check your blood level. If your blood level is normal, it is not needed. If your blood level is below normal, I suggest 1000-2000 IU daily until the low normal blood level is reached. Adjust dosage then to maintain the low normal range.

3. **Omega-3 fatty acids.** You can fulfill your daily requirement by consuming 1-2 tablespoons of flaxseed meal or 1-2 tablespoons of chia seeds each day, perhaps by sprinkling it over cereal. Be sure to refrigerate flaxseed meal.

4. **Cholesterol-lowering drugs.** These must be taken under a physician's supervision. My own preference is one of the statin cholesterol-lowering drugs, which should be started when you begin the nutrition program. Together, the drug and your new way of eating will usually reduce your total cholesterol level to less than 150 mg/dL in just fourteen days. With the help of your physician, you should monitor your progress over the first two months. I suggest three or four cholesterol measurements over that two-month period: the first and the third should be full cholesterol profiles, which includes total cholesterol, HDL, LDL, and triglycerides; the second and fourth can focus on total cholesterol alone. After two months, it is enough to have your cholesterol measured every two to three months. Why so often? This is your lifeline, giving you immediate feedback on how you are doing. If you reduce your total cholesterol to well below 150 mg/dL, you may, with your physician's assistance, reduce the drug dosage—and in some cases, eliminate it altogether.

Why not just use the diet for a number of months and add the cholesterol-reducing drug only if it is needed to force the cholesterol below the 150 mg/dL threshold? With severe coronary disease, we don't always have the luxury of time. It is essential to start the healing of the endothelium, that vulnerable inner lining of the coronary arteries, as rapidly and completely as possible. Used as adjuncts to the nutrition plan, these remarkable statin drugs help to do just that.

And there is another benefit, as well—this one psychological. As you embark on this nutrition plan, you, yourself, are in control, as Joe Crowe and Abe Brickner learned. And the empowering effects of being able to see dramatic improvement quickly, over just a matter of weeks, are impossible to overstate. You have numerical proof, in the form of radically lower cholesterol levels, that you are conquering the disease that was destroying you.

But remember: the drugs alone are not enough. In Chapter 5, I cited a study, recently reported in the *New England Journal of Medicine,* in which huge doses of statins successfully reduced patients' cholesterol levels well below 150 mg/dL. *But even so, as their diet never changed, one out of four of the subjects experienced a new cardiovascular event or died within thirty months.*

Unlike the drugs, plant-based nutrition has beneficial effects far beyond reducing cholesterol levels. It has a mighty impact on a host of other risk factors, as well: obesity, hypertension, triglyceride, and homocysteine levels. It enables the endothelium to heal and renew itself, and allows once-clogged arteries to dilate and replenish the heart muscle they serve. It makes you heart-attack–proof.

It doesn't get much better than that.

9

Frequently Asked Questions

IF YOU HAVE READ THIS FAR, you now know what you need to do. But if you're like most of my patients, you still have some serious questions. In this chapter, I will address some of the most common concerns.

Can I change?

Many patients have told me how difficult it is to change. They mention how hard it is to maintain this nutrition plan when dining with friends and relatives, during work hours, while traveling, both in the United States and abroad. But you can do it. Many others have. The key is to remember that the rewards are greater than the frustration.

I have experienced this phenomenon myself and watched it in every patient with whom I've worked: *after twelve weeks of eating no animal foods, dairy, or added oils, you lose your craving for fat.*[1] You then begin to appreciate more than ever before the natural flavor of grains, vegetables, legumes, and fruit. You develop a series of menus that you especially enjoy. Occasionally, friends get interested in what you are doing, and daringly invite you to their homes for no-fat meals. You discover restaurants that actually will cater to your needs.

You can change. While switching to a strictly plant-based diet may seem challenging at the start, all you have to do is stick with it. The satisfaction of new tastes and, above all, the health rewards make it no contest.

Will I get enough fat and protein?

The answer, emphatically, is YES.

No fat deficiencies have been identified in people who eat a variety of plant-based foods. Overall, a diet made up of the foods on the "approved" list in Chapter 8 will contain approximately 10 percent fat. That level represents a significant departure from the 37 percent fat content of the typical Western diet, but it is ideal for good health. It provides all the fat you need without giving you the extra doses that wreak such havoc with your heart health.

And this diet will not cause a protein deficiency. Typically, the Western diet contains an excess of protein—especially animal protein. The nutrition plan I recommend provides a variety of healthy plant proteins, somewhere between 50 and 70 grams every day. That is entirely adequate for a healthy lifestyle.

Could a low cholesterol level be dangerous for my health?

Some years ago, there were reports that low blood cholesterol levels might be associated with lung, liver, or colon cancer and that they might also contribute to accidental deaths and suicide. For example, one trial from Helsinki, Finland, seemed to have identified more traumatic deaths in patients using cholesterol-lowering drugs.[2]

But subsequent reanalysis of the Helsinki study and all other trials of the effects of reducing cholesterol levels, with or without drugs, have shown no increased incidence of suicide, accidents, or cancer. The newer research makes it clear that otherwise healthy individuals who achieve low blood cholesterol through proper low-fat nutrition will enhance their health, not harm it. The West Coast Family Heart Study found a reduction in both depression and aggressive hostility among those on a low-fat, cholesterol-lowering program compared to the control group eating the standard high-fat diet.[3] And in a large study from Scandinavia, patients with coronary artery disease were randomly chosen to receive either a cholesterol-lowering drug or a placebo, a harmless pill containing no medication. The members of the group that took the drug lowered their cholesterol by an average of 35 percent. After five and a half years of follow-up evaluation, they had experienced significantly fewer deaths, fewer new heart attacks, and fewer angioplasties and bypasses than those who took the placebo, and they showed no increase at all in deaths from accidents, suicide, or cancer.[4]

Will I have enough strength and energy?

If you believed all the advertisements that bombard us in print and on television, you'd think that people who didn't consume dairy and animal products couldn't possibly get the nutrients they need for strength and energy.

Nonsense. The truth is that excessive consumption of animal protein badly weakens our bodies. Among other things, it accelerates the loss of calcium through the kidneys, leading to the brittle, porous bone condition called osteoporosis. And take a look at the examples nature offers. The elephant has huge, strong bones to support its weight. Has anyone ever seen an adult elephant drinking whole milk for calcium? The muscles of an Aberdeen Angus bull are most impressive. But it is highly unlikely, to say the least, that any of those bulls have ever eaten steak.

There are plenty of examples of human athletes who achieved greatness nourished by plant-based diets. Art Still, a lean and muscular 270-pound defensive end, was convinced of the benefits of plant-based nutrition during his playing days in the National Football League. Carl Lewis, the champion sprinter, switched to a plant-based diet in the late 1980s. At the world championship track meet in Japan in 1991, at the age of thirty, he became the only man in history to broad jump farther than twenty-nine feet three times in one afternoon. At the same meet, he set a world record for the 100-meter dash and ran the anchor leg on the record-setting 4 × 100-meter relay team.

Or take the Esselstyn family. In 1984, the whole group joined Ann and me in moving toward eliminating dairy products, meats, and oils from our diet. Our eldest son, Rip, became an all-American swimmer at the University of Texas (and today is a firefighter in Austin, where his entire team at Firehouse 2 has adopted plant-based nutrition). Our second son, Ted, set a 200-yard backstroke record at Yale, and our daughter, Jane, won the Big Ten 200-yard backstroke championship while she was attending the University of Michigan. Our youngest son, Zeb, as an Ohio high school junior, was the state butterfly swimming champion. And Ann, now in her early seventies, runs between forty and seventy minutes almost every day.

You need not worry about strength and energy on my nutrition program.

What if my cholesterol won't go below 150 mg/dL?

A tiny minority of the population, no more than 5 percent of all Americans, has an inherited cholesterol disorder that makes it impossible for them to reduce total cholesterol below 400 to 500 mg/dL, even with careful nutrition. Such patients need to be monitored by highly qualified cholesterol specialists, and in rare cases, may require liver transplants to help them regain the ability to reduce cholesterol.

But for the great majority of persons, that is not a problem. So the first thing I do when people tell me that they can't reduce their cholesterol to 150 mg/dL or less is press them on precisely what they eat on Friday or Saturday nights, or what they might have consumed at that seemingly endless weekday meeting where there was "nothing else to eat." Often, under my questioning, they reveal tiny deviations from the nutrition program—lapses so small that they didn't even take them into account. One example: by the time you hold down the nozzle on a popular cooking spray long enough to coat a wok or pan, you'll build up about a tablespoon of oil. Such transgressions can easily be enough to injure the endothelium's capacity for producing nitric oxide, which in borderline cases can mean the difference between success and failure. It is that kind of attention to tiny details that makes my program work.

It is true that there are some people without heart disease who strictly adhere to a plant-based diet—no lapses at all—and even so, cannot reduce their cholesterol below 165–170 mg/dL. (Some researchers have suggested that years of eating fat and cholesterol may compromise the body's natural capacity to reduce cholesterol levels.) For these people, a modest dose of a cholesterol-lowering medication under physician supervision should take care of the problem. It is worth noting, however, that anyone who achieves a cholesterol level of 165–170 mg/dL by eating a strictly no-fat, plant-based diet is already doing wonders for his or her health, even without reaching the optimal level. That person is, by definition, consuming large quantities of natural antioxidants, which prevents the body from oxidizing LDL cholesterol into its most dangerous, artery-clogging form.

Don't my genes predetermine whether or not I'll get heart disease?

I often hear some variation on the following theme: "My eighty-seven-year-old grandfather eats nothing but eggs, bacon, cheese, and pork, and seems fine. Since I have his genes, why should I change?"

That question brings to mind an analogy: depending strictly on your genes to keep you safe while living a high-fat lifestyle is much like getting through a busy four-way intersection that has no traffic signs or stoplights; a few people will make it across unscathed, but many more will be injured—or will perish. The grandfather living on fat is obviously someone with a good cholesterol clearance mechanism and strong artery linings that resist breakdown and deposits of fatty plaque. But it is important to remember that the male grandchild asking the question does not share his grandfather's exact genetic profile. The questioner's grandmother and two parents have added to his own genetic mix, and he has no guaranteed protection against coronary artery disease as the grandfather apparently does.

I also hear the converse of that question, which is rather more to the point: "Both my father and his brother died of heart attacks at age fifty-eight, and their father had the same fate at sixty-three. Is there really anything I can do to avoid their fate? Am I condemned by my genes to have heart disease?"

This time, the answer is an emphatic NO. If you maintain a cholesterol level under 150 mg/dL, or LDL under 80 mg/dL, you—and all the other relatives who inherited these genes—will be free of heart disease. Recall, once again, the house fire analogy I ask my patients to consider. If you do not throw any fuel at all on that fire, it cannot burn.

To paraphrase William Shakespeare, the fault is not in our genes, but in ourselves and the way we eat. And that brings me to a frequently asked question that gets a chapter all its own.

10

Why Can't I Have "Heart Healthy" Oils?

DURING THE 1990S, the headlines were suddenly filled with the wonders of "the Mediterranean Diet." It was widely hailed as a much more heart-healthy approach to eating than the average American diet, largely on the basis of research by a group of French scientists headed by Dr. Michel de Lorgeril of Joseph Fourier University in Grenoble.[1] Known as the Lyon Diet Heart Study, the research spawned scores of magazine and newspaper articles and Mediterranean-style cookbooks.

For this study, the French researchers assembled 605 subjects—all of whom had survived a first heart attack—and divided them into two groups. The profiles of the two were very similar when it came to risk factors for coronary artery disease, including cholesterol and other blood lipid levels, blood pressure, and tobacco use.

About half of the subjects—302—were asked to consume a Mediterranean-style diet, which the American Heart Association defines as follows:

- High in fruits, vegetables, bread and other cereals, potatoes, beans, nuts, and seeds

- Includes olive oil as an important source of monounsaturated fat

- Dairy products, fish, and poultry consumed in low to moderate amounts, little red meat

- Eggs consumed zero to four times weekly

- Wine consumed in low to moderate amounts

Participants in this group agreed to consume a diet that averaged 30 percent of daily calories from fat—8 percent from saturated fat, 13 percent from monounsaturated fat, 5 percent from polyunsaturated fat—and just 203 milligrams a day of cholesterol.

The other participants in the study, 303 people in all, functioned as a control group, and were given no particular dietary advice beyond being asked by their physicians to eat prudently. On average, they ate a diet that the American Heart Association describes as "comparable to what is typically consumed in the United States." It derived about 34 percent of its calories from fat—12 percent from saturated fat, 11 percent from monounsaturated fat, and 6 percent from polyunsaturated fat—and included about 312 milligrams a day of cholesterol.

After a little more than a year, the researchers noted that those following the Mediterranean-style diet were doing much better than the control group. The results, they reported, were "striking." After nearly four years, the results were clearer than ever. Those on the experimental diet were 50 to 70 percent less likely to experience all the cardiac ailments the researchers recorded, from minor events that required hospitalization to major emergencies such as angina, stroke, or heart failure, to heart attacks and even death.

Impressive results. It is not surprising that they received such great attention and that the Mediterranean diet attracted many adherents. And it is also not surprising that many of my patients are at first puzzled by the fact that my nutrition plan does not permit monounsaturated oils such as olive oil or canola oil to be part of an arrest and reversal program for coronary artery disease. Because of the Lyon Diet Heart Study, the media have taken to referring to these oils as "heart healthy."

Well, nothing could be further from the truth. They are not heart healthy. Between 14 and 17 percent of olive oil is saturated, artery-clogging fat—every bit as aggressive in promoting heart disease as the saturated fat in roast beef. And even though a Mediterranean-style diet that allows such oils may slow the rate of progression of coronary artery disease, when compared with diets even higher in saturated fat, it does not arrest the disease and reverse its effects.

Dr. Walter Willet, a professor of public health at Harvard, has written a book touting the benefits of monounsaturated oil. Recently, when he was lecturing in Cleveland, I asked whether he had seen any evidence that a diet rich in monounsaturated oils has arrested and reversed coronary artery disease. No, he replied—but added that there was indirect evidence of arrest and reversal in the Lyon Diet Heart Study.

But let's take another look at that study. There is no question that the group consuming the Mediterranean-style diet did not fare nearly as badly as those in the control group. But there is another way to look at the results of the Lyon Diet Heart Study. *By the end of the study, nearly four years after its start, fully 25 percent of the subjects on the Mediterranean diet—one out of four—had either died or experienced some new cardiovascular event.*

I feel these are wretched results for a nonmalignant disease. We can do much better. During a panel discussion at the 2nd National Summit on Cholesterol and Coronary Artery Disease, in 1997, Colin Campbell, author of the best-selling China Study, was asked his thoughts on the results of the Lyon Diet Heart Study, and to compare those results with those he found in studying health and nutrition in rural China, where coronary disease is practically nonexistent. Colin didn't hesitate for a moment. The Mediterranean and rural Chinese diets are practically the same, he replied. "I would say the absence of oil in the rural Chinese diet is the reason for their superior success."

In fact, the medical literature is filled with evidence of the harmful effects of monounsaturated oil. The late Dr. David H. Blankenhorn of the University of Southern California School of Medicine compared baseline angiograms with one-year follow-up angiograms in persons with coronary artery disease. He found that the disease had progressed just as much in those consuming monounsaturated fats as it had in those eating saturated fat.[2]

Similarly, Lawrence Rudel of the Wake Forest University Baptist Medical Center experimented with the diet of the African Green monkey, which metabolizes fats very similarly to human beings. At the end of five years, he found that those monkeys consuming monounsaturated fat did show higher levels of HDL (good) cholesterol and lower levels of LDL (bad) cholesterol, but autopsies on them showed that they had developed just as much coronary disease as those fed saturated fat.[3] Rudel later repeated the experiment using rodents and obtained the same result.

Robert Vogel, the University of Maryland School of Medicine researcher whose experiments I recounted in Chapter 5, found that eating bread dipped in olive oil reduced the dilation in the brachial (forearm) artery that is normally seen with the brachial artery tourniquet test.[4] This suggested temporary injury to the endothelial cells, compromising their ability to produce nitric oxide. And Japanese researchers have shown that monounsaturated fat elevated blood sugar and triglycerides in rodents with a diabetic tendency.[5]

And once again, I invoke my own experience. In the summer of 2004, I had a call from the Reverend William Valentine of North Carolina. In 1990, he had undergone a quintuple coronary bypass. Since that surgery, he had been carefully following a plant-based nutrition program. His weight had fallen from 210 pounds to a trim 156, which he had maintained over the years. But by mid-2004, he was experiencing a recurrence of angina, especially when he exercised, and sometimes even while resting.

He had read about my program in a health newsletter, and he wanted my advice. He was extremely anxious about undergoing any repeat bypass surgery or intervention, and wanted very much to avoid it. But he couldn't imagine what more he could do, on his own, to curb the angina. And since he was eating whole grains, legumes, vegetables, and fruit, I was initially baffled.

At a loss for suggestions, I asked the Reverend Valentine to tell me, once again, everything he was eating, and to leave out absolutely nothing. This time, he added to the list. He had forgotten, he said, to mention that he was consuming "heart healthy" olive oil at every lunch and dinner and in salads.

It was what they call a Eureka moment. Immediately, I advised him to give up the olive oil. He did—and within seven weeks, his angina had completely disappeared.

11

Kindred Spirits

T. Colin Campbell, the Cornell University professor who directed and cowrote *The China Study,* observes that there are "two worlds" of medicine—two radically different visions of how to approach health. "One consensus favors drugs as the cure, the other favors food," he explains; Western medicine, for the most part, has chosen drugs. As he sees it, we got it wrong.

I agree. However, over the last couple of decades there has been some movement in the West toward recognizing the importance of nutrition to health. That is a development to be welcomed. And I much admire all the pioneers who have dared to stand up to the establishment. Their work has nourished my own, and although we may disagree on some fine points, for the most part we represent different paths up the same mountain.

Colin Campbell himself is one of these pioneers. He went to Cornell planning to study how to make more and better milk and meat protein. Once there, however, he discovered—through his own research and that of others—that those products were disastrous to human health. And with the sort of intellectual honesty that is much too rare in this age, he quickly switched his focus to follow where the science led. The *New York Times* called his *China Study* the "grand prix" of epidemiological nutrition research. He is utterly fearless, candidly analyzing the backroom deals and politics of a paranoid animal food industry that will stop at nothing to maintain the dominance of its products in the American diet. And he has played what is almost certain to be a critical role in the future of how we eat. For years, he has taught America's foremost course in undergraduate nutrition, and his students will form the foundation of American nutrition in the twenty-first century.

Nathan Pritikin is another example of those who have bravely bucked the nutrition establishment. I never met him, but I did read his books and over the years, I have worked with some whom he trained. Pritikin was an engineer who had a lifelong interest in medicine and nutrition. In the course of his studies, he learned about the Tarahumara Indians of northern Mexico, whose diet consisted almost entirely of complex carbohydrates and who suffered from almost no heart disease or cancer. Pritikin became convinced that these Indians set an example Americans should follow, and devoted much of his life to spreading that message. The diet he promoted emphasized consumption of vegetables, fruits, whole grains, and small amounts of meat, poultry, and fish—all told, a low-fat, high-fiber diet supplemented with healthy doses of aerobic exercise.

Because Pritikin did not have a degree in medicine, his research was never fully accepted by the medical community. Even so, he never backed down, and ably defended his viewpoint against his critics. Proof that he had been on the right course all along came after his death in 1985, at the age of sixty-nine, of complications from experimental treatment for leukemia. The *New England Journal of Medicine* published the results of his autopsy, noting an "absolutely remarkable" absence of calcification and fatty deposits in Pritikin's coronary arteries. Those blood vessels, the medical examiner declared, were like those of a teenager.[1]

Hans Diehl, who studied with Nathan Pritikin, has made healthier lifestyles his own lifelong cause. His Coronary Health Improvement Program—CHIP—trains entire communities in how to change their bad nutrition habits. I have been one of CHIP's guest speakers on numerous occasions and have experienced firsthand the magical influence its founder can have in mobilizing large groups of people to take control of their own health.[2]

Yet another pioneer in the field is a physician named John McDougall, who for more than thirty years has been teaching about the critical importance of diet to health. I read his book *The McDougall Plan* in 1983, and it helped convince me that I was on the right track in my own growing belief in plant-based nutrition. Dr. McDougall became interested in the subject when he lived in Hawaii, on a sugar plantation. As he tells the story, "I met first-, second-, third-, and fourth-generation Filipinos, Japanese, Chinese, and Koreans." He noticed that his patients from the first generation of immigrants, who ate the "worst diet," according to traditional nutritional principles—virtually no dairy products or meat—always seemed trim and fit. "They avoided heart disease, diabetes, breast cancer, prostate cancer, and arthritis, by and large, and they also lived to work and function fully into their eighties and sometimes nineties on a diet primarily of rice and vegetables." But as the succeeding generations became more Westernized and learned to eat what the experts considered a "well-balanced diet," they became fatter and sicker. "This caused me to reevaluate everything I was taught previously about 'good nutrition,'" says Dr. McDougall. Ever since, he has been writing and teaching about the benefits of a primarily vegetarian, "starch-based" diet. Joel Fuhrman, a board-certified family physician in New Jersey, has long been a strong advocate of plant-based nutrition. He has vigorously promoted his health message throughout this country and is the author of two excellent books: *Eat to Live* and *Disease-Proof Your Child*.

Of all the low-fat nutritional programs that have emerged over the past twenty years, perhaps the most similar to mine is that of Dean Ornish. I have known Dr. Ornish for twenty years, and I have the greatest respect for his work. At my invitation, he has spoken at the Cleveland Clinic and at national conferences on preventive cardiology. Among the wide variety of programs promoting cardiovascular health, his and mine are the only ones I am aware of that are based on peer-reviewed research that demonstrates arrest and reversal of heart disease.

As you have read, my own twelve-year study started in 1985. I set a clear goal: achieving total cholesterol in my patients of less than 150 mg/dL using a plant-based diet and cholesterol-lowering medication. The emphasis was on absolute adherence to my nutritional program, which I reinforced through my interviews with patients and my reviews of their diet diaries every two weeks for the first five years, every four weeks for the second five years, and every twelve weeks for the last two years of the study. All of the participants in my research were severely ill, with disease in all three-coronary arteries. Most had undergone a previous heart bypass operation or an angioplasty that eventually had failed. Several had failed these procedures twice. And several had been told by their cardiologists that there was nothing further to be done—that they must prepare for the inevitable progression of their disease.

Following earlier groundbreaking studies, Dr. Ornish began another study in 1986. Like mine, his aimed to reverse coronary artery disease through plant-based nutrition. But he did not specify cholesterol targets for his patients, and he did not use cholesterol-reducing medication. Like mine, Dr. Ornish's patients had three-vessel coronary artery disease. And Dr. Ornish insisted that in addition to adopting a plant-based diet, his patients must use relaxation and meditation techniques and participate in a structured exercise program. Finally, Dr. Ornish had a control group of patients who had similar disease severity, but who followed a traditional program of cardiac care.

My own research had convinced me that it was plant-based nutrition, rather than meditation or exercise, that protected people in certain cultures from developing coronary artery disease, so I did not require anything of my patients apart from an absolute commitment to eat according to the plan. I wanted them to focus absolutely on proper nutrition, and I worried that asking them to make too many changes in their lifestyle would interfere with that focus. Since the health benefits of relaxation and exercise are well documented, they were free, of course, to meditate if they chose to (none did) and I encouraged them to exercise (most chose walking—although there was an occasional jogger or swimmer). It is worth noting that two of my patients, who had had moderately disabling strokes before the study began, did no exercise at all—yet like the others, they had excellent results that have lasted more than twenty years since the start of the study. Patients with coronary artery disease who cannot exercise must not despair. Full adherence to the nutrition program will protect them from progression of their disease.

Just one year into his study, Dr. Ornish published his findings to date. During those first twelve months, his experimental patients had suffered less severe and less frequent attacks of angina than the members of the control group. Follow-up angiograms had showed reversal of coronary artery disease among the experimental group, and that benefit continued at the five-year follow-up study. Additional PET-scan imaging of his experimental patients at five years confirmed that 99 percent were able to halt or reverse disease. There was a direct correlation between adherence to the program after one year and after five years.

Dr. Ornish reported twenty-five new coronary events in his experimental patients at five years, which were 2.5 times fewer events than were identified in his control patients receiving traditional cardiac care. I have personally met some of Dr. Ornish's original patients, who like mine were doing well nineteen years later. The Ornish program has been expanded to multiple sites throughout the nation.

I waited five years before publishing my first report on our results. Angina was diminished in all patients, and had completely disappeared in several more. Follow-up angiograms had shown some stunning reversals of disease. Average total cholesterol was 137 mg/dL, and average LDL was 77 mg/dL. After twelve years, the end of the formal study, I could report that seventeen of the eighteen original patients had experienced *no* subsequent coronary events since the start of the research. (One noncompliant patient had required bypass surgery.) And more than twenty years later, as I noted in Chapter 6, these patients continue to flourish.

To the best of my knowledge, the twelve-year report on my patients represents the longest follow-up study in the medical literature of arrest and reversal of coronary heart disease.

The key, as both Dean Ornish's research and mine clearly show, is in persuading patients to grasp the total message and to comply fully with the programs. Our approaches differ in some significant ways, but the goal is the same: stopping heart disease in its tracks and even eradicating its effects.

And what of future generations? There has been some significant progress on that front, as well.

It started with the publication, in 1995, of *Dr. Attwood's Low-Fat Prescription for Kids: A Pediatrician's Program of Preventive Nutrition.*[3] This wonderfully comprehensive book observed that by the age of twelve, 70 percent of American children have fatty deposits in their arteries, the precursors of heart disease. In his book, Dr. Charles Attwood, who died in 1998, destroyed many of the common myths about the harmful effects of plant-based eating for children and adolescents. Among them: the notions that a child on a plant-based diet won't attain full growth or have enough energy, that he or she won't consume enough calcium, protein, and iron, that controlling obesity and cholesterol can wait until the child is older. Not one of these premises is true.

A longtime pediatrician with an extremely busy practice, Dr. Attwood felt an obligation to eliminate the barriers that prevent children from exposure to healthy low-fat eating. Most significant, he took a very courageous step in recommending the elimination of dairy products, meat, fish, fowl, and oil from the pediatric diet—recommendations accepted and endorsed by the late Benjamin Spock, who wrote the foreword for Attwood's book. Since the book was published, similar advice has proliferated in bookstores and on the Internet, and today it does not seem so revolutionary to suggest that providing children with low-fat, plant-based nutrition will protect them from the ravages of heart disease and the common cancers in their adult years.

But will children develop a taste for healthy eating?

Antonia Demas answers that question with a resounding yes. During the 1990s, while pursuing her doctorate in nutrition at Cornell, Demas performed a controlled experiment in Trumansburg, New York. Her subjects were children from kindergarten through fourth grade who prepared, cooked, and consumed a plant-based diet. She was able to show that when introduced to the subject of nutrition in a hands-on learning process, children not only adopted healthy, low-fat diets—they did so with enormous enthusiasm. Her doctoral thesis based on that research, *Food Education in the Elementary Classroom,* won numerous awards and international attention.

Demas now heads the Food Studies Institute, a nonprofit organization, based in Trumansburg, which is devoted to the long-term health and education of children. In 2001, she published *Food Is Elementary,* an elementary-school curriculum that uses a multidisciplinary approach to teach children about food, nutrition, culture, and the arts. In addition, Demas's institute works with schools across the country to incorporate low-fat, high-fiber choices into school meal programs and to get parents involved in what their children are learning about nutrition.

I take great pleasure in all these developments. And yet, with all the research that demonstrates the wisdom and benefits of plant-based nutrition, its growing ranks of proponents still face a formidable array of opponents, from the titans of the animal food industry to the medical establishment itself. My colleague Dean Ornish succinctly sums up the dilemma faced by those of us who believe in this healthy way of eating: "I don't understand why asking people to eat a well-balanced vegetarian diet is considered drastic, while it is medically conservative to cut people open."

Well said.

12

Brave New World

HEALTH CARE, to put it mildly, is an industry out of control. If we don't make some major changes, projections show that by the year 2014, spending on health will account for nearly one-fifth of America's gross domestic product.[1] By the middle of this century, spending on Medicare alone will consume an estimated 40 percent of the U.S. budget. This is unsustainable, and its effects are already showing up in a variety of painful ways.

Even as I write, General Motors—once the biggest, most powerful corporation in the entire world—is announcing draconian plant closings and workforce cuts that will eliminate more than 30,000 jobs in North America over the next few years. The main reason is the cost of health care for GM's current and retired workers, which is now so high that it adds $1,500 to the price of every vehicle the company manufactures. And General Motors is hardly alone. Starbucks, one of the most successful companies of the past two decades, recently announced that it is spending more on health care for employees than it spends on coffee beans.

Across the American economic spectrum, employers are trying desperately to rein in health costs, asking workers to pick up more of the tab for their care or, in many cases, dropping insurance coverage entirely. Labor unions are discovering that they cannot negotiate contracts that keep wages apace with inflation because the cost of health care is severely eroding corporate profit margins. Companies are closing down factories and jobs at home and relocating them overseas, where wages and health costs are much lower. All the while, increasing numbers of American workers are sliding into the ranks of the uninsured.

What can we do? I have a fairly radical answer for that question: *We should aim at eliminating chronic illness.* That is not an unattainable goal.

Most of America's health dollars are spent on the late stages of heart disease, strokes, hypertension, diabetes, and the common Western cancers of the breast, the prostate, and the colon. Like heart disease itself, these others are part of the bitter harvest of the toxic American diet. And like traditional treatments for heart disease, their treatment is not preventive. Having your breast cancer amputated, your malignant prostate gland radically removed, or your cancerous colon resected is painful, disfiguring, and costly—and too often does not resolve the underlying problem.

My own research has concentrated on coronary artery disease, and how plant-based nutrition can prevent and also arrest and reverse it. But with every year that passes, there is more proof that a plant-based diet has similar salutary effects on other chronic diseases, as well.

Take stroke, for example—the third leading cause of death in the United States. The evidence is overwhelming that if you eat to save yourself from heart disease, you eat to save yourself from stroke.

There are two types of stroke. In hemorrhagic stroke, the less common of the two, a blood vessel in the brain ruptures because of high blood pressure or a genetic weakness of the vessel wall known as an aneurysm. A plant-based diet cannot do anything to cure a genetic aneurysm. But it will definitely help reduce blood pressure, an important step in the right direction.

On the more common variety of stroke—ischemic or embolic stroke—there is even better news. These have the same origin as coronary artery disease. An ischemic stroke occurs when fat and cholesterol block blood vessels that carry oxygen and nutrients to the brain, just as they may block the coronary arteries that nourish the heart. An embolic stroke also deprives the brain of nutrients and oxygen, but in a slightly different way. When an artery sheds part of its diseased inner lining, that debris—called an embolus—is carried through the bloodstream until it gets wedged into a blood vessel that is too small for it to traverse. Now it blocks the flow of blood through that vessel. This may happen almost anywhere in the body, blocking blood flow to a kidney, an intestine, a leg, or some other organ. When it occurs in vessels that nourish the brain, it is a stroke.

In the 1990s, Pierre Aramenco, a physician from Paris, studied this process in Frenchmen who were at risk for vascular disease.[2] Using ultrasound probes inserted through the esophagus, Dr. Aramenco measured the thickness of atherosclerotic debris growing on the inside of each patient's ascending aorta, the giant artery that climbs directly from the heart and sends branches to the brain. He divided the men into three groups. One group showed 1 millimeter of debris on the lining of the aortic wall. The second had debris measuring between 1 and 3.9 millimeters thick. The third had more than 3.9 millimeters of debris. Dr. Aramenco followed the patients for three years. Not surprisingly, the group with the greatest amount of plaque growth shed the greatest number of emboli, and had the most strokes (see Figure 17 in insert).

The buildup of fatty plaques in blood vessels can cause damage in many different ways. For example, when an aorta that contains plaque is clamped during coronary bypass surgery, plaque debris is loosened and enters the bloodstream as an embolus. Using ultrasound to monitor the middle cerebral artery in the brain, technicians can distinctly hear the embolizing plaque as it enters the brain. If the patient dies during surgery, the plaque debris may be found in the brain at autopsy.

This tragic sequence helps explain the fearful loss of cognition in coronary artery bypass patients.[3] But neuroradiologists also report that using magnetic resonance imaging, they can detect little white spots in the brains of Americans starting at about age fifty. These spots represent small, asymptomatic strokes (see Figures 8 and 19 in insert). The brain has so much reserve capacity that at first these tiny strokes cause no trouble. But, if they continue, they begin to cause memory loss and, ultimately, crippling dementia. In fact, one recently reported study found that the presence of these "silent brain infarcts" more than doubles the risk of dementia.[4]

We now believe, in fact, that at least half of all senile mental impairment is caused by vascular injury to the brain. Not long ago, a Swedish study of five hundred eighty-five-year-olds found that fully one-third of them showed some form of dementia. A careful analysis revealed that in half of those with dementia, their mental impairment was due to a diseased arterial blood supply to the brain.[5] Similarly, a study in the Netherlands focused on five thousand people between the ages of fifty-five and ninety-four.[6] The researchers studied the circulation in the brains of all their subjects, then asked them to perform various written tests of mental acuity. The results were quite clear: those suffering from artery disease and thus impaired circulation in the brain performed less well on the tests than did those whose arteries were clean. Age made no difference. Arterial health was the variable that counted.

This should come as no surprise. Clogged arteries serving the brain and clogged arteries serving the heart are part and parcel of the same disease. The cause is the same: a buildup of fat and cholesterol and lethal damage to the delicate endothelial lining of the blood vessels. And the cure is the same, as well: adopting a healthful new way of eating that includes not a single ingredient known to damage vascular health.

Just as you are not doomed to heart disease as you grow older, you also are not doomed to mental deterioration. Most cases of stroke and dementia, like heart disease, need never occur. Your aorta, along with all your other arteries, can be as clean at ninety years of age as they were when you were nine.

Two of my original heart patients had strokes before joining my nutrition program. William Morris had just one stroke. Emil Huffgard had three. As a result, both had suffered impairment of their walking. More than twenty years later, both of these men are alive and well. Neither has had any further strokes. The same plant-based nutrition that saved their hearts also saved their brains.

I have mentioned previously that several of my patients have also noted a distinct improvement in their sex lives. And recent research confirms a strong connection between impotence and cardiovascular disease. In December 2005, researchers reported on a study that followed 3,816 men with erectile dysfunction and 4,247 without over seven years.[7] It turned out that the men who were impotent before the study began or who developed it during the study were 45 percent more likely to experience a cardiovascular event than

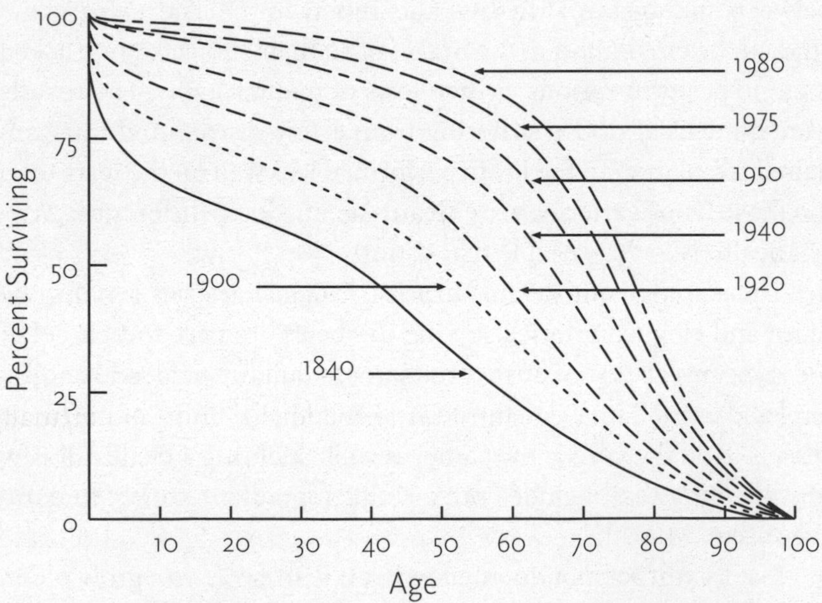

Figure 20. Survival curves, 1840–1980, reveal that our life expectancy has greatly increased but our life span has remain unchanged. (Reprinted with permission from Vitality and Aging: Implications of the Rectangular Curve.*)*

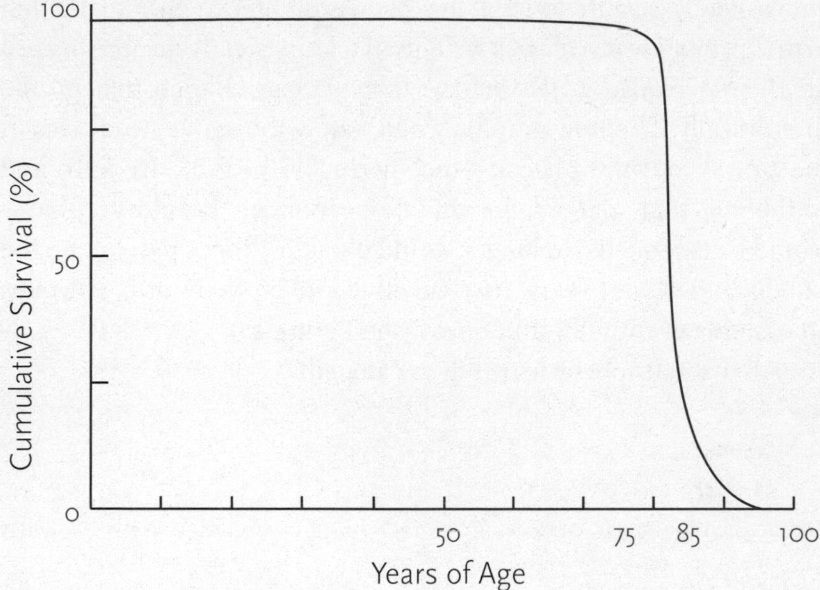

Figure 21. If we are to shift the survival curve significantly to the right, for a rectangular survival curve, we need to overcome chronic diseases. (Reprinted with permission from Vitality and Aging: Implications of the Rectangular Curve.*)*

those free of erectile dysfunction. Impotence, it turns out, is as robust a predictor of cardiovascular disease as elevated cholesterol, smoking, or a strong family history of the disease. Our own anecdotal evidence suggests that profound lifestyle change with plant-based nutrition offers the optimal opportunity to avoid heart disease—and to restore erectile capacity.

With every passing year, we understand more about the mechanisms through which nutrition affects our health, and virtually everything we are learning underscores the benefits of abandoning the high-fat habits of old in favor of a plant-based diet that fills our plates and our selves with a most nutritious array of disease-preventing, injury-healing, health-enhancing ingredients.

If you were to chart the course of most people's lives in the modern West—as explicated by Dr. James Fries and Dr. Lawrence Crapo in a book entitled *Vitality and Aging*[8]—the graphic would show steady health toward the prime of life, a period on that prime plateau when all was well, then a long, steady decline toward death (see Figure 20). I believe that we can change that profile dramatically. The new graphic would show the same steadiness in the prime, but the plateau—that period of health, strength, and well-being that marked the middle section of the old graphic—would be extended. No longer would chronic illness precipitate the sad decline of later years. Instead, all would be well until, naturally, all systems eventually shut down (see Figure 21).

All that, simply by learning to eat well.

13

You Are in Control

WHEN I JOINED the Cleveland Clinic's staff in 1969, locker room space in the senior surgical staff dressing room was at a premium. Locker assignments were alphabetical, and as my last name begins with an *E*, I was assigned to double up with a doctor whose name began with *F*. For two years, René Favaloro and I shared the same surgical locker.

Dr. Favaloro, a native of Argentina, was a brilliant, creative, and compassionate surgeon. In May 1967, he started a revolution in cardiac surgery. He cut out the blocked portion of a patient's right coronary artery, then replaced it with a small piece of vein from the patient's leg. In September of that same year, he performed the first true coronary bypass surgery, sewing a piece of vein into the ascending aorta, then tapping it into the coronary artery below the blockage. Over the following years, he developed many variations to the bypass surgery approach, and today is universally recognized as the creator and innovator of that type of surgery. I have often thought about the irony here—how two surgeons sharing the same locker could end up approaching coronary artery disease from such diametrically opposite positions.

But perhaps Dr. Favaloro and I were not so much at odds, after all. Not long before his death in July 2000, Dr. Favaloro himself described "an unreasonable gap between the medical enthusiasms devoted to acute interventions and the meager efforts currently devoted to secondary prevention."[1]

There will always be special situations in which patients with unstable coronary artery disease will require some type of urgent bypass or intervention, but I am convinced that with improved nutrition, we can spare a growing majority of patients from these procedures. And I am pleased to see that quite a number of scholarly cardiologists are beginning to question the wholesale rush toward mechanical intervention in heart disease.

One of them is Dr. John Cooke of Stanford University, who readily acknowledges that angioplasty—while it can help to relieve angina—hardly ever saves lives, and does nothing whatsoever to cure heart disease. He suggests, in fact, that about half of all angioplasties performed in the United States each year are simply unnecessary. Dr. Cooke writes: "In my opinion, it is far better, and well within your ability, to restore the health of your endothelium rather than have a cardiologist remove it with a balloon catheter. If your doctor recommends angioplasty, tell him or her that if at all possible, you prefer a medical and dietary approach. Angioplasty should be reserved for emergency situations (when someone is in the middle of a heart attack) or when medical and nutritional therapy have been attempted but failed to relieve the symptoms."[2]

Similarly, Dr. James Forrester and Dr. Prediman Shah of Cedars-Sinai Medical Center in Los Angeles have criticized the fact that cardiologists are so quick to intervene with angioplasty or bypass procedures. In their own research, they wrote: ". . . we are led to the remarkable conclusion that angiography does not identify, and consequently revascularization therapies do not treat, the lesions that lead to myocardial infarctions."[3]

In June 2005, researchers who conducted a meta-analysis of 2,950 cases of coronary artery disease reported in the journal *Circulation* that in patients with chronic, stable disease, intervention "does not offer any benefit in terms of death, myocardial infarction or the need for subsequent revascularization compared with conservative medical treatment."[4] And a year later, Dr. Richard Krasuski of the Cleveland Clinic's top-rated cardiology department said flatly that aggressive treatment of patients with stable angina is generally unwarranted. "We don't prevent heart attacks or death," he declared. The reason: "Heart attacks can begin in any heart artery, not just those highly blocked vessels treated by angioplasty or stenting. So in general, the best prevention is control of risk factors that can protect every vessel in the body."[5]

The thesis of my research has been absurdly simple: using a plant-based nutrition program to reduce cholesterol to the levels seen in cultures that never experience heart disease. My patients were willing in 1985 to put their cardiovascular health in the hands of a general surgeon who told them this was an illness that did not exist in three-fourths of the earth's population. If it could be arrested and reversed in monkeys, I told them, it could also be arrested and reversed in humans. They decided to join in my experiment.

Our research data have clearly confirmed that we were right. My patients' decision to enter the study not only put an end to the progression of their disease; the information we have gleaned from their experience has set a new gold standard in the therapy for coronary artery disease. We can arrest and reverse it. We can make ourselves heart-attack–proof. *Coronary artery disease need not exist, and if it does, it need not progress.*

The argument I still hear from physicians who do not embrace this truth is that they are certain their patients would not comply with such a strict nutrition program. I do not understand how they are so sure of this unless the patients are given a chance; in fact, after counseling patients with severe coronary artery disease for more than twenty years, I have found the opposite to be true.

If you explain to a cardiac patient that there is a program that will quickly relieve or eradicate his pain, that can eliminate any need for further intervention—no more bypass surgery, angioplasties, or stents—that can heal and replenish the vascular system, that has benefits that improve over time, the patient tends to pay attention. In my experience, in fact, like that distraught man on the cruise ship who heard me lecture—"I can't believe no one told me there was another option!"—many thoroughly resent the fact that no one ever told them the truth.

Patients who undergo bypass surgery have, on average, a 2.4 percent chance of dying and another 5 percent chance of sustaining a stroke or heart attack during the procedure. Four percent of patients who get stents have heart attacks during the stenting, and 1 percent die. Let's put flesh on that statistic: since there were more than 1 million stent operations last year in the United States, that means 40,000 patients had heart attacks during the procedure—and 10,000 died. If 10,000 American soldiers died in one year in Iraq, it would be called carnage. As the late Cleveland Clinic urologic surgeon William Engel said, "It is acceptable to lose an occasional patient, but best not to hasten them along."

One of my recent patients had a terrifying experience with interventional cardiology. In September 2004, Jim Milligan, an insurance executive from Wooster, Ohio, was helping his wife can tomatoes. Suddenly he began to sweat and felt considerable chest pain. He sat up all night, the pain constant. The next day, at his wife's insistence, he went to a local emergency room, where he was told he was having a heart attack.

Jim was rushed by ambulance to a hospital in Columbus for an urgent angiogram, which revealed significant blockages in his coronary arteries. A doctor inserted a catheter in order to put a stent in place. Suddenly, Jim couldn't breathe. He had "a terrible taste" in his mouth. He started shaking. He was experiencing anaphylactic shock, a life-threatening reaction to the dye used for the angiogram. The procedure was immediately terminated, and Jim spent five days in intensive care.

Over the next four months, cardiac nuclear scans revealed that the blood supply to Jim's heart was deteriorating. His left ventricular ejection fraction—the measurement of the heart's capacity to pump blood, which is normally above 50 percent—was down to 40 percent.

In January 2005, Jim called me. It was apparent in his counseling session that he entirely grasped our message. And over the next four months, his cholesterol plummeted—from 244 mg/dL to 140 mg/dL. His body weight fell from 254 pounds to 204. His longtime cardiologist wanted him to return to Columbus for an additional angiogram and, likely, more stents, but Jim was adamant about sticking to the arrest-and-reverse program. He found another cardiologist who did some research on me and was supportive of what Jim was trying. "If Dr. Esselstyn says do something," he told Jim, "I'll work with you."

By April 2005, tests revealed that Jim's left ventricular ejection fraction had returned to 62 percent—normal. He was given a clean bill of health, with no restrictions on his activity and, perhaps more important, given his anaphylactic scare, no further need for intervention.

It is difficult to imagine a patient with coronary artery disease, facing an elective intervention, who would not respond when told the truth about the dangers of the procedure. Reminded that the surgery will relieve only the symptoms of the illness, wouldn't almost anyone choose, instead, to treat the underlying disease through arrest-and-reversal therapy?

Patients want to avoid the potential complications and mortality involved in intervention. Those who are sent home to die by their cardiologists, after failing bypass or stents, rejoice as they lose weight, lose their angina, lower their blood sugars, decrease their dose of insulin or come off it altogether, reduce the use of medication, see stress tests revert to normal, diminish the plaque plugging their arteries, and resume a fully active life. They are visibly empowered by the knowledge that they, not their physicians, now have control over the disease that was destroying them.

Even those who may be dubious at first are often won over. Several years ago, I encountered a doctor from Pittsburgh who had been advised at his own hospital to undergo bypass surgery but was reluctant to do so. He sought a second opinion from an eminent cardiologist at the Cleveland Clinic, who finally talked him into having a stent. The surgery was performed, but the stent was unsuccessful. The Pittsburgh doctor knew about my program, but declined to participate, fearing that it would cramp the active social life he and his wife enjoyed at home. He found that by reducing his activity, he could live within the limits of his angina.

Seven months later, I called to see how he was doing. Not surprisingly, he was still imprisoned by the chest pain. Frustrated on his behalf, I raised my voice over the phone: "Gordon, for God's sake, just give me sixteen days and I will get you out of prison." He agreed.

After sixteen days, his angina was almost gone—and it disappeared entirely over the following two weeks. That doctor is now a fierce advocate of my program, a complete believer in plant-based nutrition.

And here is something that gives me great pleasure—and a good deal of hope: these days, more patients are coming to me *before* they go through interventional procedures. And when they adopt the profound lifestyle changes I demand, they are finding that the interventions are no longer necessary.

John Oerhle is a case in point. John is a man who has never allowed a physical handicap to stand in his way. When he was sixteen, he was making a bomb in his basement and ended up blowing off his right hand and all but two of the fingers on his left. Nonetheless, he went to MIT and became a highly successful aeronautical engineer, as well as a croquet champion and top bridge player.

In 1993, after his brother had a heart attack, John started seeing a cardiologist who prescribed medication that he would have to take for the rest of his life. Ten years later, he experienced shortness of breath. He failed a stress test, then had an angiogram, which revealed 80 percent blockage of two major arteries and 100 percent blockage of a third. Not surprisingly, he was scheduled for open-heart bypass surgery.

Once onboard that train, it takes an unusual person to step off. But John *is* unusual. The scientist in him was too strong. He read widely on his disease, and ultimately canceled the surgery. Online, he Googled "atherosclerosis reversal therapy"—and found my website. He and his wife, Catheryn, came to see me and immediately grasped what I was recommending.

Within a month after he committed himself to plant-based nutrition, John Oerhle's total cholesterol dropped to 96 mg/dL, and his LDL—bad cholesterol—to 34 mg/dL. One year later, after another stress test, John's cardiologist commented: "I'd be hard-pressed to say there is anything wrong with this heart."

Then there's the case of Dick Dubois, a chronic marathoner and president of a container recycling facility in New York State. In the fall of 2004, Dick began to experience occasional tightness in his chest during his training runs. A stress test showed nothing abnormal, and he continued running. But the pain worsened, and by February 2005, an echo stress test suggested a partial blockage of the right coronary artery. His doctors prescribed cholesterol-reducing medication, aspirin, and a beta-blocker. But the pain persisted. He began walking, instead of running. Even so, through the summer of 2005, he continued to have chest pain.

In September of that year, an angiogram revealed multiple blockages in Dick's coronary arteries. The worst was an 80 percent blockage at the origin of the left circumflex and left anterior descending artery. Dick's cardiologists were concerned that any attempt at angioplasty or stenting could be fatal, and they scheduled an appointment for a bypass procedure with a leading cardiac surgeon at the Cleveland Clinic.

As it happened, shortly after the angiogram Dick had read *The China Study,* T. Colin Campbell's brilliant work on nutrition and disease. He was interested in the chapters that described my work, and ultimately contacted me. On October 9, 2005, Dick and his wife, Rosalind, came to Cleveland for counseling. They decided to try my approach at least until the December appointment with the heart surgeon. When the surgeon called to say there was an unexpected opening in his schedule, and gave Dick an earlier appointment on October 26, Dick thought about it, but decided to stick with our program for at least two months. By the time the surgeon called, just eleven days after our counseling session, he was no longer experiencing any chest pain during his walking workouts. Eventually he canceled the surgery, even though the surgeon warned that left untreated, he had a 10 percent chance of dying within a year.

Three weeks after the initial counseling, Dick's total cholesterol was just 101 mg/dL and his LDL (bad) cholesterol was 49 mg/dL. All his numbers looked terrific. I called him every seven to ten days to evaluate his progress. Each time, he reported new activities—cross-country skiing, then snowshoeing—which he pursued sensibly, reducing the intensity if it caused angina. In January 2006, eleven weeks after his counseling visit, Dick told me that a January thaw had made skiing and snowshoeing impossible, so he had gone to the high school track. He jogged for one mile and for the first time in more than a year he experienced no chest pain.

The stories of John Oerhle and Dick Dubois reveal how powerfully and promptly the body can heal itself from a devastating illness. And they underscore a point I have repeatedly stressed: patients with stable coronary artery disease should be cautious about the "quick fix" approach of bypass surgery and stents, which pose significant risks of complications and mortality. They should be offered intensive lifestyle change for twelve weeks in a reasonable trial. If they devote themselves to the progam with unwavering commitment, many will avoid entirely the need for surgical intervention.

I still cherish the naive dream I had when I started this research. We have shown that the number one killer in Western civilization can be abolished, through consumption of a plant-based diet. But we can do much more. If the public adopted this approach to preventing disease, if, by the millions, Americans abandoned their toxic diets and learned a truly healthy approach to eating, we could largely limit all those diseases of nutritional extravagance—strokes, hypertension, obesity, osteoporosis, and adult-onset diabetes. Meanwhile, we would see a marked reduction in cancers of the breast, prostate, colon, rectum, uterus, and ovaries. Medicine could relinquish its primary focus on pills and procedures. Prevention, not desperate intervention, would become the order of the day.

Even I am not optimist enough to believe that this could happen overnight—that the entire population of the United States would switch to a plant-based diet the moment its benefits are widely known. But we can get there. The first step is to educate the public, teaching the truth about what we know about nutrition and the ravages of the traditional Western diet.

In my fantasies, for instance, I imagine a widespread use of the brachial artery tourniquet test (BART), which Dr. Robert Vogel used to such devastating effect to prove the vascular damage a single meal can cause. If public schools were forced to serve only meals that are BART-positive (i.e., maintaining normal artery dilation), if restaurants were required to inform us which menu items are BART-positive and which are BART-negative, if the labeling on all packaged foods carried information on their BART status, we would have gone a long way toward enlightening citizens and helping them make informed choices about enhancing or destroying their health. Although my BART fantasy may never come true, the basic point is that the place to start is definitely by enlightening the public.

Then, perhaps, we can slowly put in place some institutional changes. For instance, we can approach insurance companies, employers, and representatives of labor with a modest proposition: that heart patients targeted for the mechanical intervention of bypass surgery or stenting should first try twelve weeks of arrest-and-reverse therapy—plant-based nutrition plus, where necessary, cholesterol-reducing drug therapy. In fully compliant patients, we see angina disappear in just a few weeks, and stress tests may return to normal in eight to ten weeks, so the results would be clear to everyone involved: for the great majority of patients, the dangerous, costly mechanical intervention would be rendered unnecessary.

What I am proposing would require revolutionary changes in the world of medicine. My father used to observe that as long as medicine was practiced on a fee-for-service piecework basis, comprehensive preventive medicine would never become the driving force in a physician's life. He was right. As I argued in Chapter 1, there are now no incentives built into the system to encourage the public to adopt healthier lifestyles. I once asked a young interventional cardiologist why he didn't refer his patients for a nutrition program that could arrest and reverse their disease, and he replied with a frank question: "Did you know that my billed charges last year were over five million dollars?"

This has to change. The collective will and conscience of my profession is being tested as never before. Now is the time for legendary work.

Those of us who practice medicine must engage in a new covenant with the public. We must never underestimate the layman's ability to adopt healthier lifestyles. We must tell the truth. We must relinquish the procedural focus of medicine and take pride in prevention. We must rejoice in conveying knowledge that empowers individuals to take control of their own health.

The late Lewis Thomas, a highly respected physician and revered medical philosopher, lectured at the Cleveland Clinic in 1986. He referred to the mechanical wizardry available in vascular disease—the angioplasties and bypass procedures—as "halfway technology." A mechanical approach to a metabolic, biochemical epidemic, he argued, was not the answer. Dr. Thomas further cautioned that there would be a moral and ethical challenge to physicians down the road: to relinquish this halfway technology in favor of simpler, safer metabolic and biochemical cures.

The time is now. The weight of scientific evidence and public opinion, once the truth is known, will prevail. And finally, we can start teaching people how to walk alongside the edge of the cliff, instead of desperately trying to save them after they fall off.

With this approach, the war against our most devastating diseases can be won.

PART TWO

The Joy of Eating

14

Simple Strategies

As you have already learned, my nutrition program is quite different from most others. It is not about making moderate changes to slow the progression of heart disease. It is about embarking on a significant change in lifestyle that will actually *arrest* the disease's progression and selectively *reverse* its effects.

Central to the program's success is the fact that the patients themselves assume complete control over their disease. They alone have the capacity to abolish it. They alone, in sticking with my nutrition guidelines over time, have the ability to ensure that the beneficial effects will expand and endure. They treat more than the symptoms of heart disease. They treat its underlying cause—and with it, the underlying cause of a host of other chronic illnesses.

The program's goal, to repeat, is maintaining total blood cholesterol below 150 mg/dL using a plant-based diet and, where necessary, cholesterol-reducing medication. And the key to success is attention to detail. In this program, we eliminate entirely the ingestion of all building blocks of atherosclerosis. *There are no exceptions.* Patients must erase the phrase "This little bit can't hurt" from their vocabulary and from their thinking. As we have learned, the opposite is true: every little bit *can* hurt—and does.

At this point, if you are like most of the patients I see in person, you are probably thinking something like this: "How on earth will I be able to give up cheeseburgers, French fries, steak, mayonnaise, cheese, olive oil, and all the other things I love?" One friend of mine, a lawyer, was so put off by the idea of giving up all those foods that he asked me whether he couldn't keep eating his high-fat diet until he developed symptoms of coronary artery disease—and *then* stop eating fat. I dissuaded him from this approach by explaining that in fully one out of four patients with heart disease, the first symptom is sudden death.

Still, there is no question that the high-fat diet typical of a Western lifestyle appeals to the palate. And its appeal is reinforced by the toxic food environment that surrounds us. The advertisements that bombard us feature foods with a much higher fat content than the level recommended by our government health agencies—and that recommended level itself is too high for optimal health. Culinary schools for chefs who eventually will be in charge of restaurant, hotel, and institutional cuisine do not teach them how to prepare healthful, tasty, attractive meals that contain only about 10 percent fat. Collectively, the media; the meat, oil, and dairy industries; most prominent chefs and cookbook authors; and our own government are not presenting accurate advice about the healthiest way to eat.

And it's not just a matter of bad information. The truth is that we are addicted to fat—literally. Receptors in our brains account for our addiction to nicotine, heroin, and cocaine, and similar cravings have been identified for fat and sugars, as well.

The way to break the fat habit is to abstain entirely from eating it—just as those who use heroin, cocaine, and nicotine must give them up once and for all. We have all seen what happens with many people who go on reduced-fat diets in order to lose weight. A diet that permits even a modest amount of animal, dairy, and oil fat still feeds the habit. The craving remains. And the moment the diet is completed—or, more often, fails—the dieter too frequently returns to his or her old habits of eating and regains the lost weight.

About a decade ago, the Monell Chemical Census Center in Philadelphia tested the effect the consumption of fat has on our desire for it. In the Monell experiment, healthy volunteers were separated into three groups. One group continued eating a typically high-fat American diet. The second ate a diet in which fat was reduced to 20 percent of total calories. In the third group's diet, the fat level was held to 15 percent or less. At the end of twelve weeks, the first two groups craved fat just as much as ever. But those who had eaten less than 15 percent dietary fat over that period had completely lost their desire for fat.[1]

The reason weight-loss diets fail is the same reason present cardiac rehabilitation for coronary artery disease fails: patients continue consuming fat. They may consume slightly less than they did before their heart disease was diagnosed, but this is still the very same fat that injured their arteries in the first place. Their heart disease continues to progress.

The people in my research study held their dietary fat to very low levels. (Although my nutrition plan requires no calorie counting, my research shows that a diet drawn from the recommended categories of foods holds fat consumption at 9 to 11 percent of total calories consumed.) Just like those in the Monell Center study, my patients lost their craving. After twelve weeks, they no longer felt as if they were in a constant state of denial, and they began to reap the myriad benefits of eliminating the fats from their nutrition. This is a lifestyle change that works.

Even so, I concede that it is not easy to change. In my experience, there are four primary challenges that confront those who embark on this program. Over the years, we have identified a variety of strategies to deal with each one:

1. **You are craving fat.** Have faith. As I explained above, that craving will disappear after three months of consuming

no fat. (By "no fat," I mean no animal, dairy, or oil fat—no additional fat beyond the natural amounts in vegetables, fruits, and grains.) You will develop a new taste for the natural flavors of food and you'll discover new herbs, spices, and sauces for seasoning. Eating safely in this culture is a daily challenge, but attention to detail assures success. And remember: you should beware of the "0 fat per serving" products such as salad dressing, butter substitutes, mayonnaise, and pastries. They may contain less than 0.5 grams per serving, but that little bit is enough to ensure that you will continue to crave fat. It also may increase your fat intake to more than 20 percent of the calories you consume, adding pounds of artery-clogging fat to your diet each year.

2. **You are invited out to eat at someone's home.** If the person inviting you is a close friend, this shouldn't be a problem. But if it is someone you don't know well, it can seem awkward at first. The key in this situation is candor—and, of course, basic good manners. Explain to your hosts at the time of the invitation that you follow an unusual nutrition plan and do not eat any meat, fish, fowl, dairy products, or oils. Emphasize that you would very much enjoy the pleasure of their company, and that you'd love to come, but don't want to cause any extra effort on your behalf. You might suggest that you could eat before arriving, then join the dinner party for a glass of wine. Almost always, the host will insist that you come for food, as well, and will ask what you can eat. In that case, tell him or her that you'd be happy just to partake of plain salad and bread—or that simple steamed vegetables or a baked potato would be just fine. (Perhaps this goes without saying, but you should always avoid pressing the issue of your diet on others unless they seem genuinely interested.)

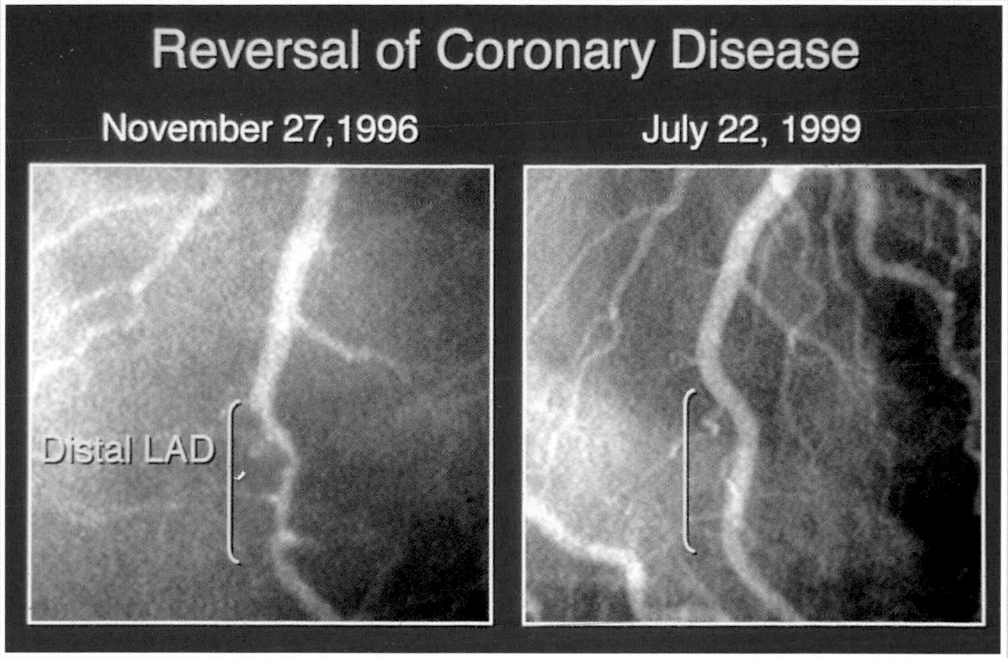

Reversal of Coronary Disease

November 27, 1996

July 22, 1999

Distal LAD

FIGURE 1 *Coronary angiograms of the distal left anterior descending artery before (left bracket) and after (right bracket) 32 months of a plant-based diet without cholesterol-lowering medication, showing profound improvement.*

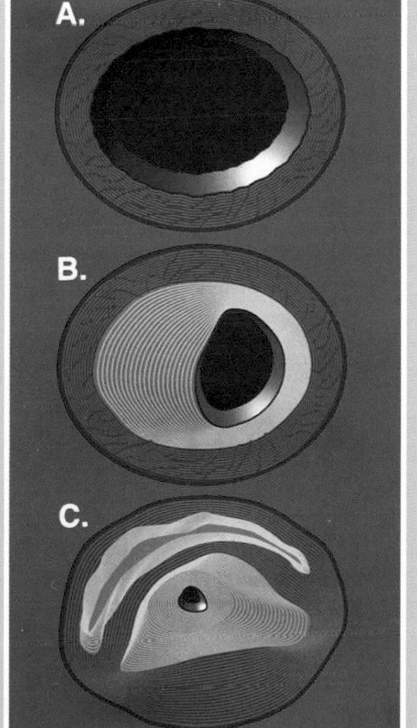

FIGURE 2 *Gradually progressive coronary artery narrowing, which accounts for 12.5 percent of heart attacks.*

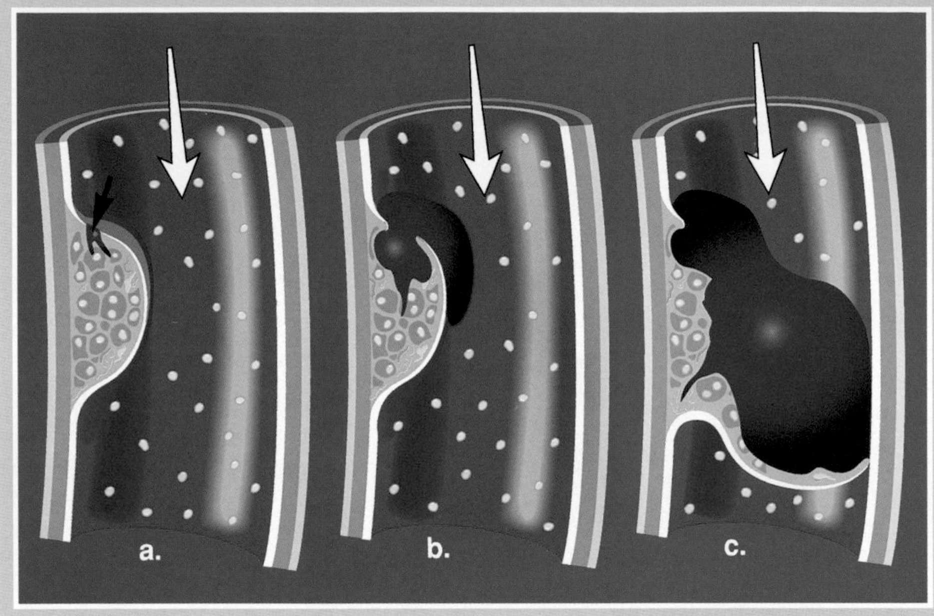

FIGURE 3 *Abrupt plaque rupture (a) with clot formation (b) and blockage (c), which accounts for 87.5 percent of heart attacks.*

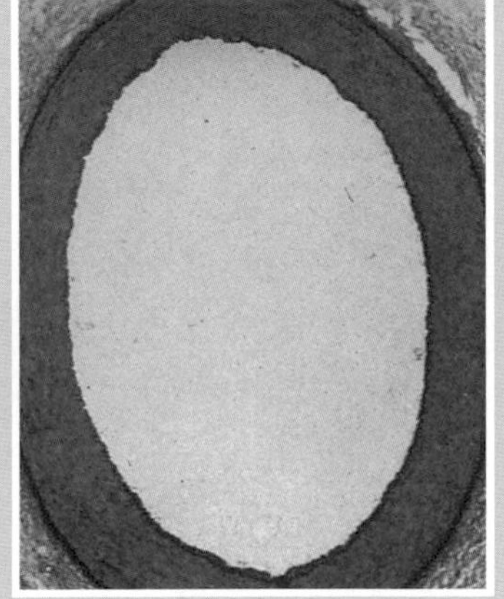

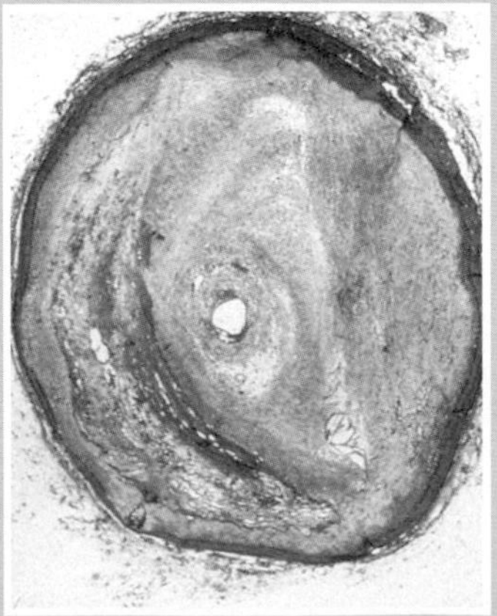

FIGURE 4 *Normal artery (top) and severely diseased artery (bottom) filled with fibrotic scar calcium, cholesterol, and fat.*

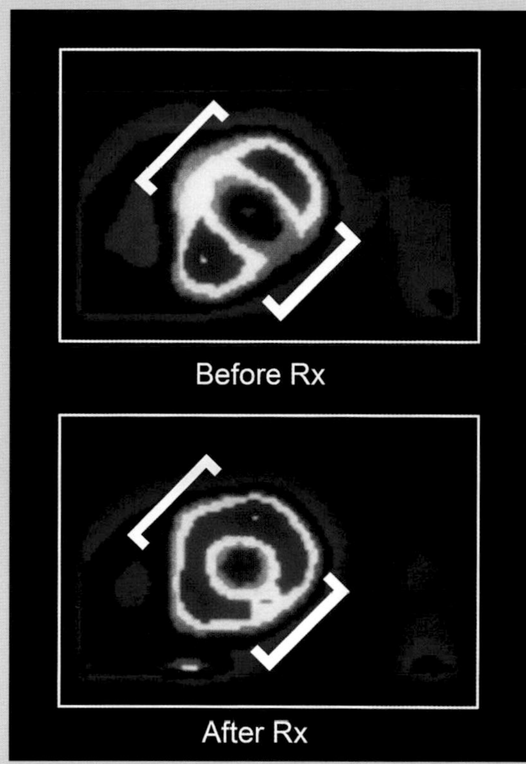

Figure 7 *(Above) Bracketed area in cardiac PET scan shows lack of blood flow. (Below) After only 3 weeks of intense plant-based nutrition, there is profound flow restoration.*

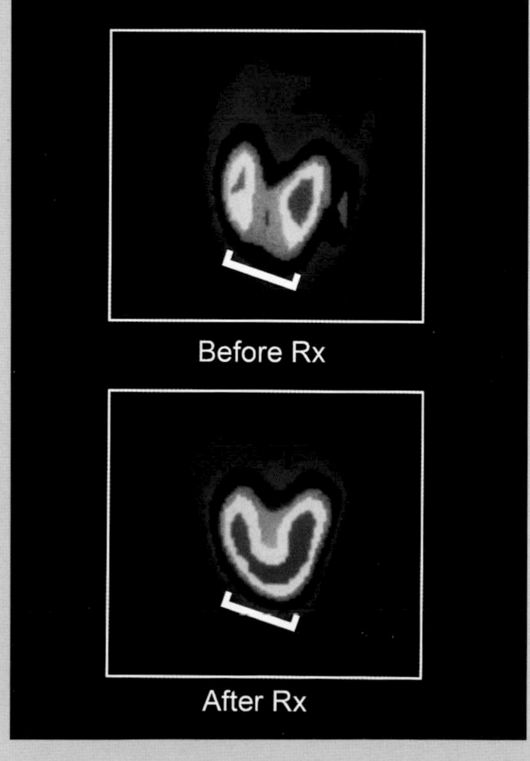

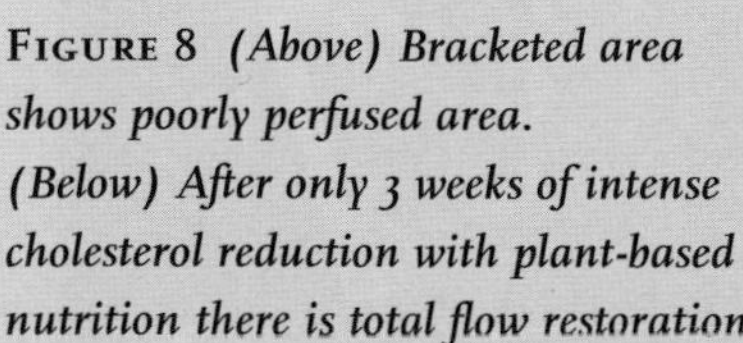

Figure 8 *(Above) Bracketed area shows poorly perfused area. (Below) After only 3 weeks of intense cholesterol reduction with plant-based nutrition there is total flow restoration.*

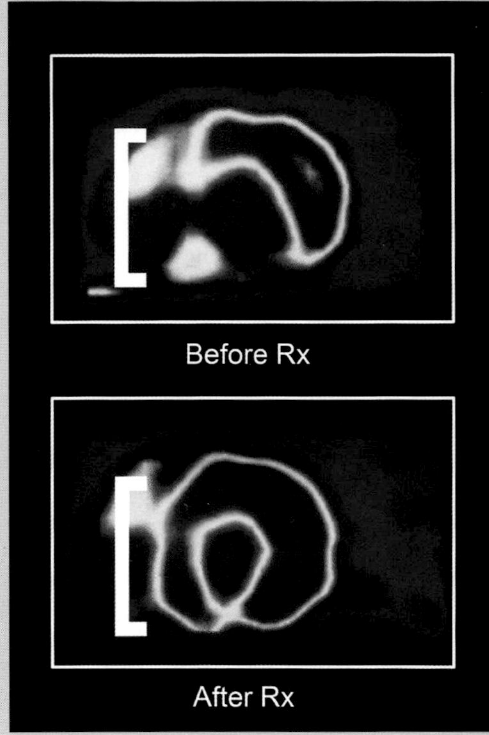

Figure 9 *(Above) Bracketed area in cardiac PET scan shows significant loss of blood perfusion. (Below) After 6 weeks of intense cholesterol reduction with plant-based nutrition there is almost total flow restoration.*

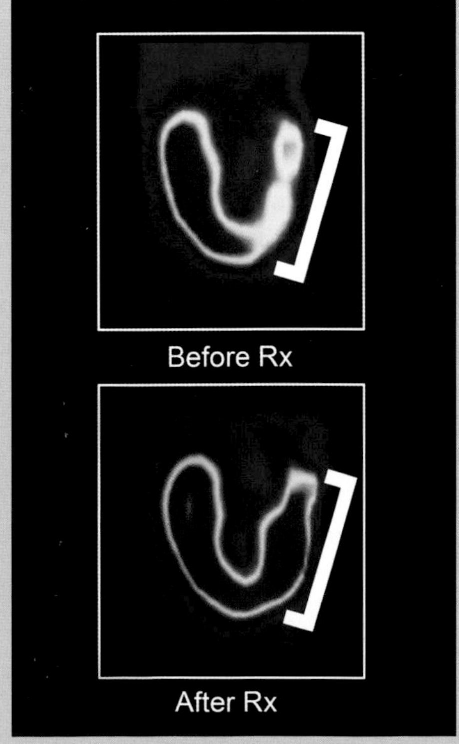

Figure 10 *(Above) Bracketed area in cardiac PET scan shows significant loss of blood perfusion. (Below) After 12 weeks of intense plant-based nutrition there is significant flow restoration.*

Figure 11 *(Above) Bracketed area in cardiac PET scan shows severe loss of blood perfusion. (Below) After 12 weeks of intense plant-based nutrition there is increased flow restoration.*

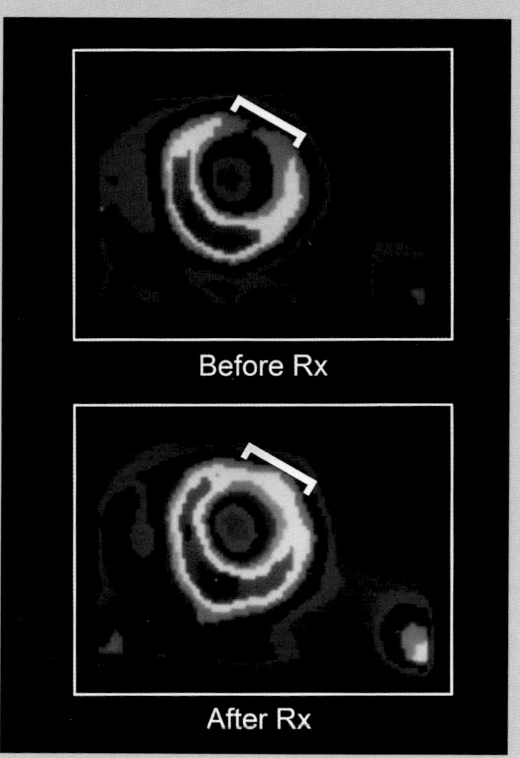

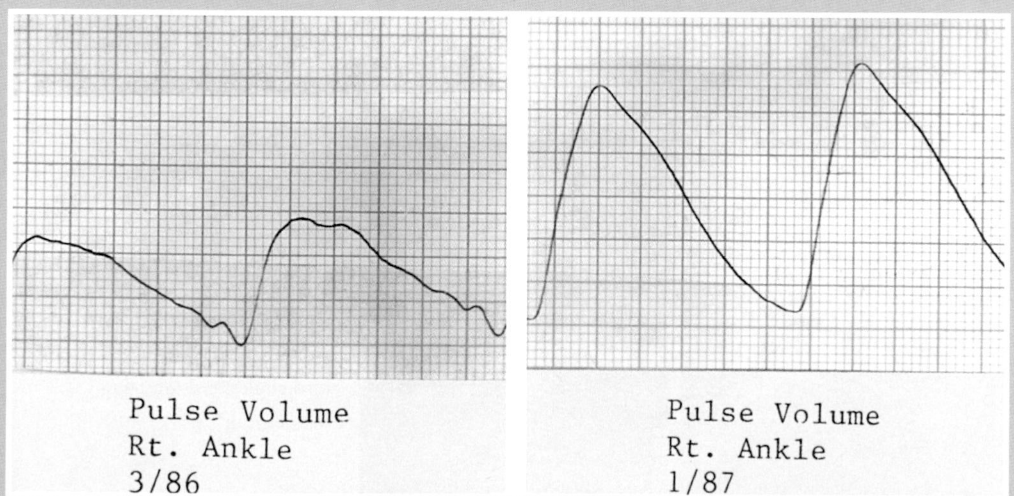

Figure 12 *Pulse volume is severely diminished (left) before therapy with intense plant-based nutrition. After therapy (right) there is full pulse volume restoration and resolution of symptoms in less than 9 months.*

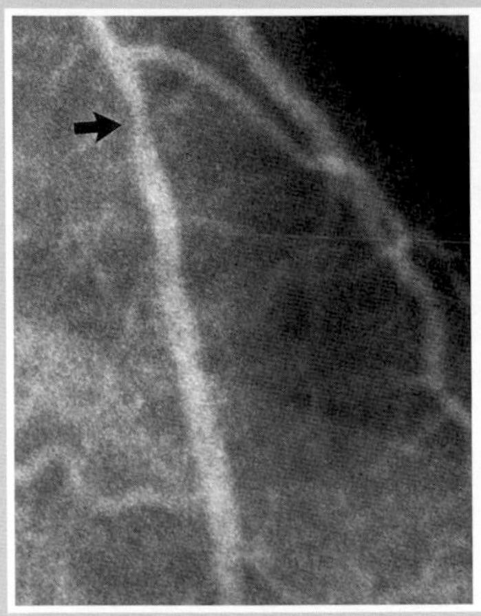

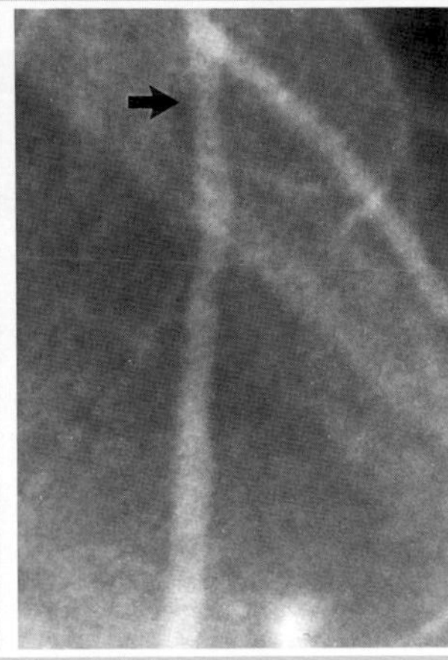

Figure 13 *Coronary angiograms of the proximal left anterior descending artery before (left arrow) and then showing 10 percent improvement (right arrow) after approximately 60 months of a plant-based diet and cholesterol-lowering medication.*

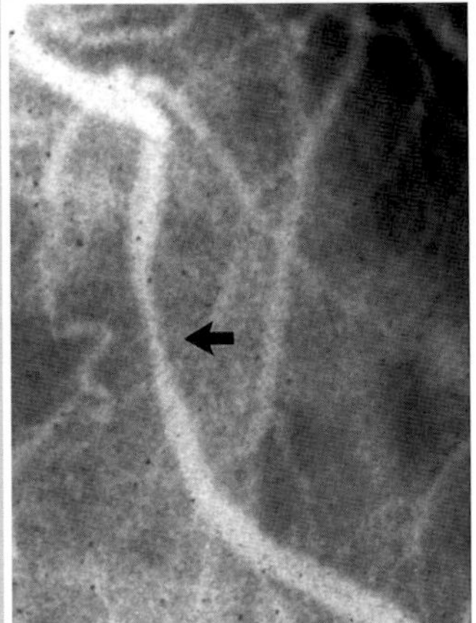

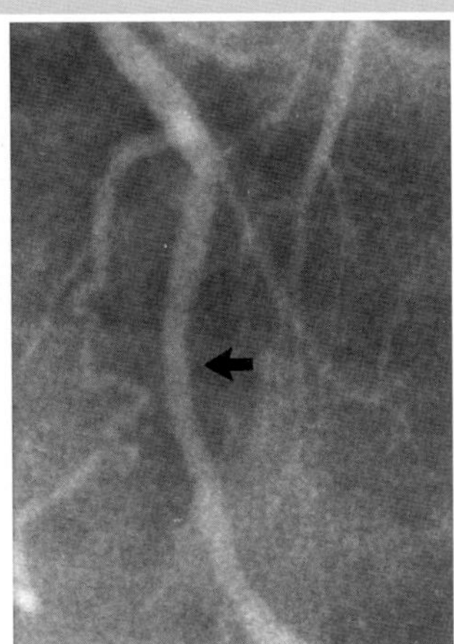

Figure 14 *Coronary angiograms of the circumflex artery before (left arrow) and then showing 20 percent improvement (right arrow) after approximately 60 months of a plant-based diet and cholesterol-lowering medication.*

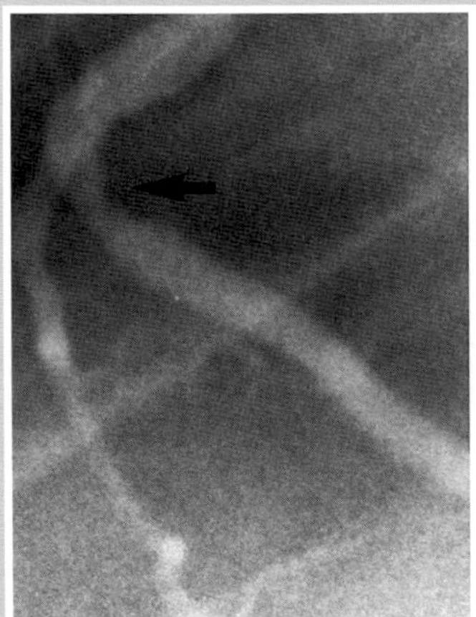

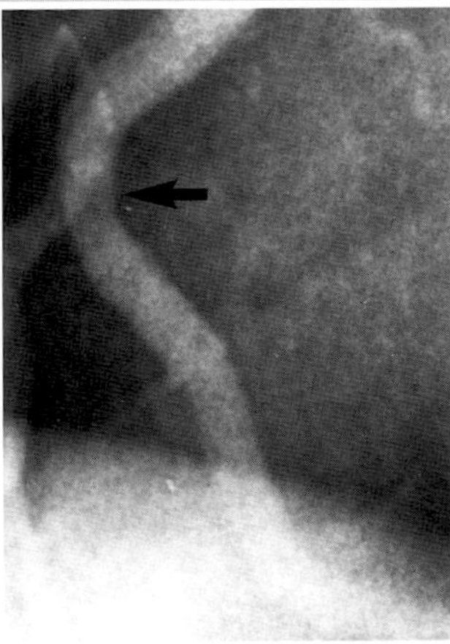

Figure 15 *Coronary angiograms of the right coronary artery before (left arrow) and then showing 30 percent improvement (right arrow) after approximately 60 months of a plant-based diet and cholesterol-lowering medication.*

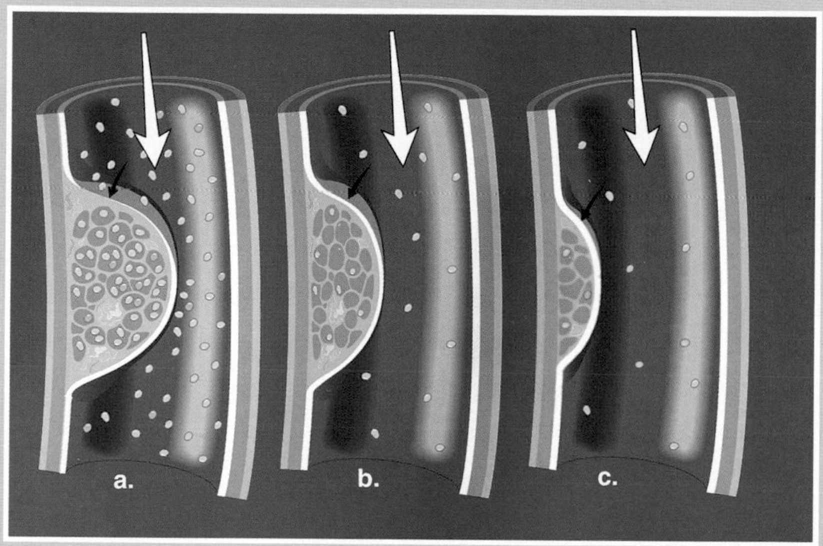

Figure 16 *Gradual plaque cap thickening (black arrow) and plaque shrinkage as achieved through plant-based nutrition.*

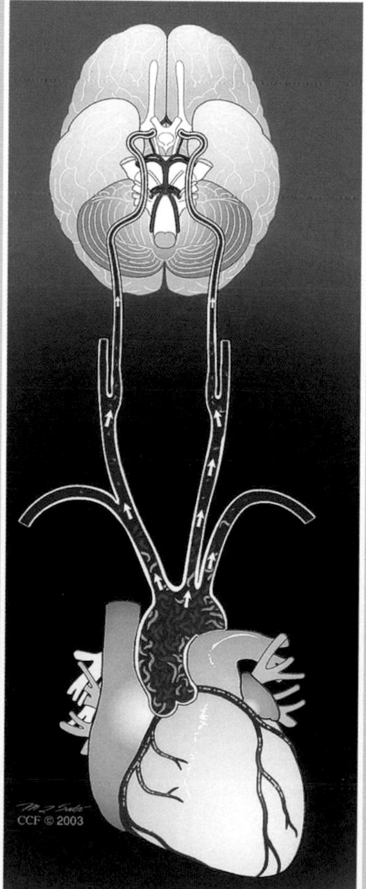

Figure 17 *Large arching vessel, or aorta, from the heart may fill with plaque debris, which in flaking off may travel, or embolize, to the brain, causing large or small strokes.*

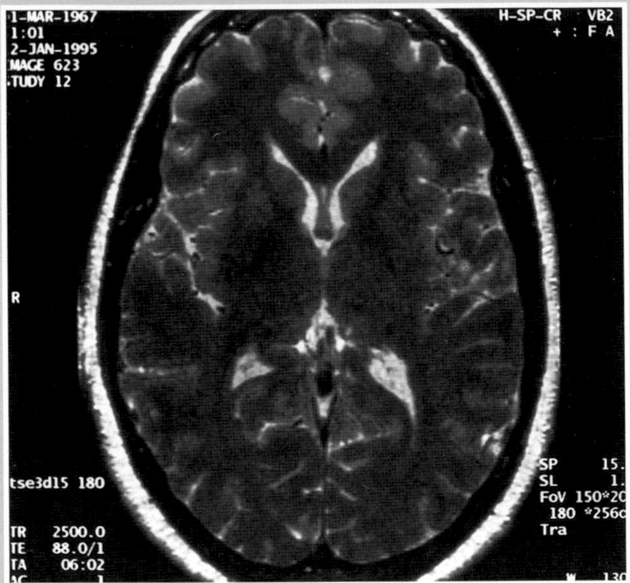

FIGURE 18 *Normal brain magnetic resonance imaging (MRI).*

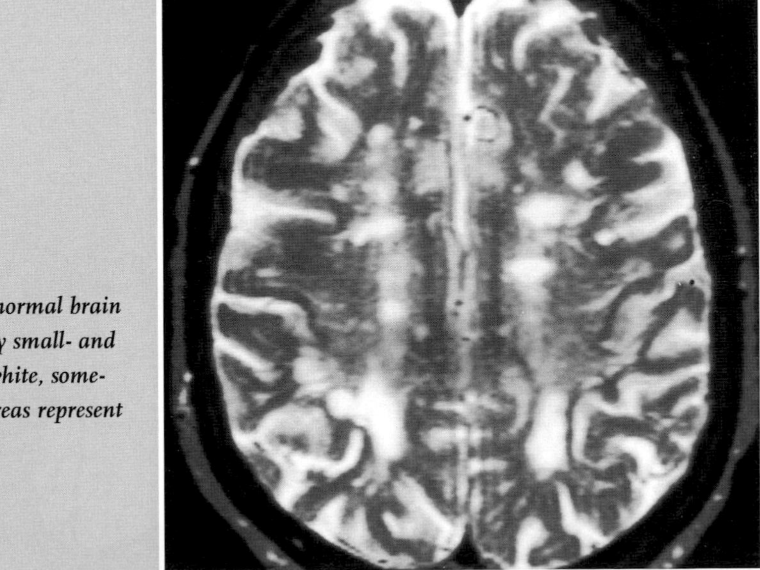

FIGURE 19 *Abnormal brain MRI—the many small- and medium-sized white, somewhat circular areas represent multiple strokes.*

3. **You must eat out in a restaurant.** Restaurants can be lethal if you don't think ahead. It is a good idea to get to know several in your area that already provide or are willing to fix a "safe" meal that you will enjoy. If you must eat in an unfamiliar restaurant, try calling the chef or maitre d' a few hours in advance—even sooner, if you have a chance. Explain that you need a meal that includes no food of animal origin, and no oil. They may well surprise you: often, restaurateurs are quite pleased to be challenged to accommodate you. And they will always be grateful that you gave advance notice.

4. **You are traveling, either at home or abroad.** Airlines can be responsive to special requests for no-fat vegetarian meals, but they often need a reminder twenty-four hours before takeoff. Of course, you always have the option of packing a picnic of your own that meets your specifications exactly. As for restaurants in unfamiliar locales, use the same tactics while traveling that you use at home: try to call ahead and let the chef or maitre d' know what kind of meal you will need.

You will doubtless come up with strategies of your own. My patient Anthony Yen, who travels far and wide on business, has shown particular ingenuity over his twenty-plus years on the program. Among other things, he put together a set of cards that request—in a variety of languages—plant-based food that contains no oil. That way, no matter where in the world he finds himself, he can confidently request the sort of meal he needs.

But if his forward planning fails, Anthony is perfectly capable of improvising. Not long ago, he went out for lunch with his son and ordered a very simple vegetable meal at a Chinese restaurant. When the food arrived, however, he could see that there was oil on it. Anthony's solution: he ordered two bowls of hot water, and washed the oil out of the vegetables. Satisfied that it now met his standards, he happily consumed the oil-free meal.

Sometimes, there's not such a ready solution. On a recent trip to the Far East, the airline forgot to load Anthony's special meal. In that case, he simply didn't eat anything but a couple of bananas on the whole twenty-hour flight. (Anthony, incidentally, mentions a side benefit to plant-based nutrition: he no longer experiences jet lag. "It used to take a week to ten days to recover" from a trip to China, he reports. "Since Esselstyn's program, I have no more jet lag." I have no scientific reason to believe that my nutrition plan is actually responsible for this, but I am happy to take credit!)

In our house, my wife, Ann, is the cook, and over the past twenty years she has learned a great deal about how to concoct wonderful meals that meet the strict standards of my nutrition plan. During the sixty- to ninety-minute counseling sessions I hold with all prospective patients and their spouses, Ann shares her own experiences and insights into how to plan and prepare dishes and menus that they will enjoy for the rest of their lives. In the following chapters, she will do the same for you. She will describe general principles and imaginative techniques that will help you put together delicious, nutritious meals for a lifetime of healthy eating.

Remember—I cannot stress this often enough—*attention to detail is the key.* If you eat in this wonderful new way, you need never develop heart disease. If you already have heart disease, you will conquer it. That is my promise to you, the sum of everything I have learned. Pay attention.

You are in control.

15

Advice from Ann Crile Esselstyn

AT FIRST, the changes you are about to make may seem overwhelming. After all, you will have to abandon the eating habits of a lifetime, and you almost surely will have to say good-bye to some beloved foods. But as we have learned from long experience, a positive attitude creates miracles. Tastes change as you eliminate the fats. Before you know it, healthy foods will be not what you *ought* to but what you *want* to eat.

As time goes by, salads with oily dressing and pizzas thick with cheese just don't seem appealing anymore. A handful of grapes or of sweet grape tomatoes becomes just as much of a treat as a cookie once was. Pizza without cheese or whole-grain bread topped with fresh, sliced peaches may well become among your very favorite things to eat.

As my husband already has stressed, it is attention to details that makes this program so powerful. But some general principles underlie the details, and it is important to understand them. Put simply, the totally plant-based diet contains:

- A fat content in the range of 9 to 12 percent of total calories consumed, none of it derived from added oils or from animal or dairy products.

- No cholesterol.

- A minimal amount of free radicals—those chemical substances that are so harmful to the body and so prevalent in the typical Western diet.

- Many antioxidants, natural compounds that neutralize free radicals and supply generous amounts of natural fiber. (Fiber has two great benefits: it is essential to health, and also helps fill you up.)

If you have heart disease—or if you never want to develop it—it is critical to grasp these absolute rules:

The rules

1. Do not eat meat.

2. Do not eat chicken, even white meat.

3. Do not eat fish.

4. Do not eat *any* dairy products. That means no skim milk, no nonfat yogurt, no sherbet, and *no cheese at all.*

5. Do not eat eggs. That includes egg whites and even egg substitutes that contain egg whites.

6. Do not use *any oil at all.* Not even virgin olive oil or canola oil.

7. Use only whole-grain products. That means *no* white flour products. Be sure the list of ingredients uses a phrase like "whole wheat" or "whole grain." Avoid semolina and wheat flour, which are actually white. Use brown rice.

8. Do not drink fruit juice. (It is fine to eat fruit, or to use small amounts of fruit juice in recipes or to flavor beverages.)

9. Do not eat any nuts (although if you have no heart disease, you can occasionally have walnuts).

10. Do not eat avocados. That includes guacamole!

11. Do not eat coconut.

12. Eat soy products cautiously. Many are highly processed and high in fat. Use "light" tofu. Avoid soy cheese, which almost always contains oil and casein.

13. Read *The China Study,* by T. Colin Campbell with Thomas M. Campbell II (BenBella Books).

Keeping these rules in mind, the rest of the world of vegetables, legumes, and fruits is yours to enjoy, and it's a very rich world, as you will learn.

A few words about salt: we do not use it. And we do not include it in our recipes, since most of my husband's patients have cardiovascular disease and hypertension, and salt may cause further injury. We have found that most patients readily adjust to the natural flavor of a plant-based diet without salt.

If you miss salt, try vinegar, lemon, pepper, Mrs. Dash (in a variety of blends), Tabasco, or other hot sauces. If you *still* miss salt, try adding a little Bragg Liquid Aminos (available in health food stores), South River Sweet White Miso, or low-sodium tamari. Try to limit sodium consumption to less than 2,000 mg a day. Your choices are easier when you know the salt content of various seasonings. Some useful comparisons:

- Sea salt, 1 teaspoon: 2,360 mg sodium

- Low-sodium tamari, 1 teaspoon: 700 mg sodium

- Bragg Liquid Aminos, 1 teaspoon: 233 mg sodium

- South River Sweet White Miso, 1 teaspoon: 115 mg sodium

It is helpful to keep breakfast and lunch simple—and nearly the same every day. Specific recipes follow in the chapters ahead, but there are lots of useful ways to think about putting them together. For example, great basics for breakfast include cereals such as old-fashioned rolled oats, a brand of shredded wheat with no added sugar, or a product such as Grainfield's raisin bran. You can top the cereal with Grape-Nuts for crunch. You might also add raisins, a banana, or other fruit. A bit of apple juice, cider, or fresh orange or grapefruit juice (include the fruit sections) is delicious in place of milk. But you can also eat your cereal with milk, oat milk, almond milk, or nonfat soy milk. And cereals are far from the only breakfast option. Pancakes made from whole-wheat flour (containing no eggs and no oil) are really good! Toasted whole-grain bread topped with summer-ripe, fresh peaches heads my own list of outrageously delicious breakfasts. You should also try sliced bananas, ripe mangos, strawberries, or other favorite fruits on toast. Think outside the box. Why not breakfast on lentil or pea soup or—my personal favorite—leftover salad?

Start as many meals as possible with salads. They're healthy and filling, and satisfying in a wonderful way. Add all the vegetables you can. Salad dressing can be a bit difficult at first, now that you are eating no oils at all. It is important to find one that you like, so spend some time experimenting. We have come to like salads dressed simply with a combination of balsamic vinegar and hummus that does not contain tahini (which is high in fat). We've found two good commercial varieties of fat-free hummus—one from Sahara Cuisine and the other by Oasis Mediterranean Cuisine (see Appendix I)—or you can make your own, using chickpeas, lemon, and garlic. Mixed with a bit of lemon or lime juice or vinegar and a little mustard, it makes a marvelous dressing.

Try to keep lunch simple: salad, soup, and bread or sandwiches. For the last, think creatively. Food for Life makes a widely available no-fat wrap (under the brand name Ezekiel 4:9), and you can spread it with no-fat hummus. Fill the hummus-spread wrap with any combination of ingredients that appeals to you: chopped cilantro, green onions, shredded carrots, cucumbers, tomatoes, peppers, thawed frozen corn, beans, rice, cooked broccoli, mushrooms, spinach, or lettuce. Roll it up into a sausage-like shape, cut it in half, put it on a baking sheet and bake at 450 degrees for about ten minutes, until the wrap is crisp. Fabulous!

At dinner, we highly recommend another healthy salad and a variety of fresh vegetables when they are in season. But there are many other options. Portobello mushrooms baked in the oven or on the grill with any barbecue sauce or low-sodium tamari and a little balsamic vinegar are wonderful and look like a piece of meat. They are great as "burgers," too, on whole-wheat bread or in buns made by Ezekiel.

Our own first and favorite dinner recipe is black beans and rice. We use it for guests, since it is beautiful to look at and almost everyone likes it. The ingredients: black beans from a can, brown rice, chopped tomatoes and their juice, chopped onion, frozen corn thawed in hot water, chopped red, yellow, or green peppers, grated carrots, water chestnuts, chopped cilantro and arugula, low-sodium tamari, and salsa. Cook the rice. Heat the beans. Put all the chopped veggies into individual dishes. Spoon rice onto your plate, pile it high with your selection of ingredients, and top with tamari and/or salsa. Store any leftovers in a bowl and use them for salad the next day, adding balsamic vinegar. Heaven!

Sometimes, the simplest foods taste the best. You can bake Vidalia onions, covered, on low heat. The longer they bake, the sweeter they become. Eat them plain or on rice or baked potatoes. Sweet potatoes and yams are delicious and filling and incredibly easy. All you have to do is remember to put them in the oven early enough, since they take at least an hour to bake. Another meal that's delicious, simple, and fast—even pretty—is whole-wheat couscous with Muir Glen's portobello mushroom pasta sauce and frozen peas. Add the couscous to boiling water and watch while it transforms itself in seconds! Heat the pasta sauce and pour it over the couscous. Thaw the peas under running water and spoon them decoratively around the sauced couscous. Instant dinner!

Much of the food you eat on this nutrition plan will be fresh vegetables and fruits, legumes, and whole grains. But there are also packaged products that can add flavor and variety to your cuisine (see Appendices I and II for suggestions and resources). Many of them are safe and delicious. However, closely examine the labels. More specifically: *Read the ingredients.*

If you see any of the following words or phrases on a label—glycerin, hydrogenated, partially hydrogenated, mono or diglycerides—avoid the product. These are all sneaky forms of fat. Snackwell's devil's food "fat-free" cookies list 0 grams of fat on the nutritional chart required on all packages. But if you read the ingredients, you notice that glycerin is listed fifth among them. Similarly, Kraft's zesty Italian fat-free dressing and Wishbone's fat-free ranch both list soybean oil and dairy products among their ingredients. But because the portion sizes are small, these products can still be called "fat-free," under the government's standard (less than 0.5% fat per serving). *Read the ingredients.*

A company called Edward & Sons makes fat-free brown rice snaps in a variety of flavors (onion garlic, tamari sesame, and unsalted) with no oil. But beware! The same company makes toasted onion and vegetable rice snaps with safflower oil added. *Read the ingredients.*

Even if you think you are familiar with a product, be careful not to get complacent. Grape-Nuts, for instance, are free of oil. So Grape-Nuts flakes probably are as well, right? Wrong! They contain vegetable oil. Avoid them. Guiltless Gourmet makes baked unsalted yellow corn chips that have no oil. But all the rest of the Guiltless Gourmet baked chips have safflower oil added. *Read the ingredients.*

When it comes to grains, you should eat only whole-grain products. There are many familiar whole grains: whole wheat, bulgur wheat, whole oats, whole rye, barley, buckwheat, whole corn, wild rice, brown rice. There are also less well-known choices: kamut, quinoa, amaranth, millet, spelt, teff, triticale, grano, faro. But it is often difficult to figure out which grains are whole and which are not. Color is not a clue; whole oats are light in color, for instance, and refined flours can be darkened with molasses.

Here, again, examine labels closely. Look for "100 percent whole." Products described as multigrain, cracked wheat, seven-grain, stone-ground, 100 percent wheat, enriched flour, or degerminated cornmeal are *not* whole grain. Pumpernickel is made with rye and wheat flours, but is seldom whole grain.

It can also be a challenge to find whole-grain bread that contains no oil or high fructose corn syrup. Great Harvest Bakery makes a number of breads that are perfect, and many grocery store rye breads have no oil. Ezekiel 4:9 sprouted grain breads are in the frozen foods section of most health food stores and an increasing number of regular supermarkets, and they come in many forms—from sliced loaves (especially good toasted), to tortillas and delicious hamburger or hot dog buns. *Read the ingredients.*

There are three cooking implements that we have found indispensable. One is a rice cooker. You put in rice and water and simply walk away; the rice cooks on its own, worry-free, and you can even start it early. The second is a microplane, which you can find at any good kitchen store. It makes the work of zesting fruit not only easy but fun. (And here's a tip on zesting: use organic oranges, limes, and lemons.) The third is a citrus reamer, which gets juice out of the driest lemons and limes. The wood ones are my favorite.

Finally, a few words about how much you should eat.

If you are eating a plant-based, no-oil, whole-grain diet filled with leafy greens and all the colorful vegetables, you don't need to worry about weight. No calculations or calorie counting will be necessary. Almost everyone loses weight with the diet change. However, if you let whole grains, starchy vegetables, and desserts dominate, weight can begin to creep back. If that happens, simply cut back on grains and starches, increase your consumption of leafy greens and colorful vegetables, and cut out desserts.

And remember, exercise does count. The more you can do, the better. For the years I taught, I managed to run (often in the dark in the winter) and to lift weights (usually before school). Now I luxuriate in having time for yoga classes, running or cross-country skiing, and some weight lifting. Essy swims a mile a day, lifts weights, and bikes three times a week. Walking, taking stairs—just moving will make a difference. It benefits the immune system, helps protect against strokes and heart attacks, osteoporosis, and dementia, inhibits cancer growth, and, of course, keeps weight down.

The basic message is simple—and welcome to so many who have battled weight all their lives: when you eat a plant-based, no-oil, whole-grain diet your body will find its own ideal weight. You will *never* have a weight problem.

Let your appetite be your guide!

16

Breaking the Fast

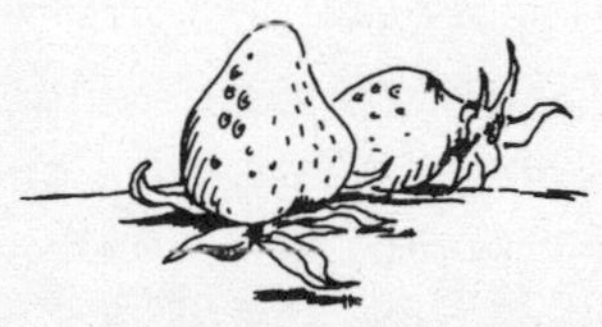

EAT BREAKFAST. Eat breakfast even if you never have before. You will have more energy and you'll avoid early afternoon hunger. Eventually, everyone develops a personal favorite.

We have discovered that many of Essy's original patients have eaten the same thing every morning for nearly twenty years. Don Felton *never* misses 1/4 cup of oat bran and 1/4 cup of quick-cooking oatmeal cooked in the microwave with water for 3 minutes, then topped with Equal. Evelyn Oswick has also eaten the same breakfast for twenty years. She calls it her "best meal of the day."

Evelyn's Best Meal of the Day

1 banana
1 cup old-fashioned rolled oats
raisins
apple juice

Slice banana into the bottom of a microwave-safe bowl. Add 1 cup oats to bowl. Sprinkle raisins over top and add apple juice to cover.

Zap it in the microwave for 1 minute 30 seconds.

Anthony's Oatmeal and Vegetables

Anthony Yen includes vegetables in his daily breakfast.

1 cup old-fashioned rolled oats
2 cups water
3 handfuls fresh spinach, or 2 cups frozen mixed vegetables
low-sodium tamari (optional)

Put oats, water, and spinach in a big microwave-safe bowl. Cover and cook 4–5 minutes in the microwave. Top with tamari.

The Esselstyn Breakfast

Our children took the family breakfast recipe with them when they went off to college. To this day, we run across friends of theirs who eat our breakfast, as do their children. A bonus: it is usually possible to find all the ingredients no matter where you travel.

1. Start with commercial old-fashioned rolled oats (not quick-cooking oats), uncooked, either plain or topped with Grape-Nuts for crunch or with another cereal like Grainfield's Raisin Bran or shredded wheat (with no sugar added).
2. Instead of milk, use oat, almond, or nonfat soy milk. Apple juice, cider, and orange or grapefruit juice (include the sections) are also delicious.
3. Top it all with raisins, sliced bananas, blueberries, strawberries, raspberries, or peaches.
4. If you don't have heart disease, add some walnuts.

Jeff's Oatmeal

Jeff is a recent patient who says he never gets tired of his oatmeal.

1. Put 1/2 cup old-fashioned rolled oats in a bowl. Sprinkle a handful of raisins over oats.
2. Add a dash each cinnamon and nutmeg.
3. Slice a medium banana on top.
4. Warm 2/3 cup of apple juice to finger temperature. Pour apple juice over the oatmeal mixture, cover, and let sit for 20 minutes. Stir and eat!

Bernie's Breakfast Salad Drink

Bernie came from Florida to learn how to eat from us, and treated us to his favorite breakfast drink—modified a bit since he invented it (it used to include almond butter and avocado). Bernie's five children grew up with this as their breakfast.

romaine lettuce
cucumber, peeled and cut in chunks
chopped celery
tomatoes, cut in chunks

Put everything in a blender or food processor and blend until smooth. Drink as is or add a little balsamic vinegar.

Larry's Sunday Buckwheat Pancakes

Larry and Ann Wheat own the famous vegan Millennium Restaurant in San Francisco. Every Sunday at home Larry makes these pancakes. Ann puts fruit on hers. He eats his with maple syrup. We even like them plain!

MAKES 12 MEDIUM PANCAKES

1/2 cup buckwheat flour
1/2 cup old-fashioned rolled oats
1/2 cup cornmeal
1 teaspoon baking powder
1/2 teaspoon baking soda
1 ripe banana
2 tablespoons vinegar
3 tablespoons maple syrup (optional)
2 cups oat, almond, or nonfat soy milk

1. Mix buckwheat flour, oats, cornmeal, baking powder, and baking soda in a bowl.
2. Mash the banana in another bowl, and add vinegar, maple syrup, and milk. Stir and add to dry ingredients.
3. Heat a nonstick pan on medium high. When water sizzles on the pan, it is ready for the pancakes. Cook until bubbles form. Flip, cook another few minutes on the other side, and enjoy eating plain or with fruit or maple syrup.

Note: If you like thicker pancakes, use less milk. And if some of the recipe is left over, make muffins. Add raisins and bake in a 350-degree oven for 20 minutes.

Barley Oat Pancakes

Top with fruit and this is almost our Esselstyn breakfast.

MAKES ABOUT 12 PANCAKES

1 cup barley flour
1 cup old-fashioned rolled oats
1 tablespoon baking powder
2 cups oat, almond, or nonfat soy milk
1 teaspoon vanilla extract

1. Mix dry ingredients in a bowl.
2. Add liquid ingredients until blended. Add water if batter is too thick.
3. Heat a nonstick pan on medium high. When a drop of water sizzles on the surface, the pan is ready for the cakes, which you can make any size you wish. After bubbles form on the top of a pancake, flip it over. Cook until underside is brown.
4. Top with fruit, applesauce, maple syrup, powdered sugar, or cinnamon.

VARIATIONS:

1. After the first pancake side starts to cook, but before the top bubbles, add blueberries, sliced bananas, or any fruit to the uncooked side, then flip until both sides are cooked.
2. For banana pancakes, use 1 cup oat, almond, or nonfat soy milk and 1 cup banana "milk" (blend 1 ripe banana, 1 cup water, 1 teaspoon vanilla extract). Mix dry ingredients with wet.

Banana French Toast

MAKES 5 SERVINGS

½ cup oat, almond, or nonfat soy milk
1 ripe banana, cut up
1 tablespoon nutritional yeast flakes (optional)
1 teaspoon vanilla extract
pinch of ground nutmeg
5 slices whole-wheat or whole-grain bread

1. Whirl first five ingredients in a blender until smooth, then pour into a shallow bowl.
2. Dip both sides of bread in mixture.
3. Cook on a preheated nonstick griddle until browned on both sides or on a nonstick baking sheet in a 400-degree oven, turning once, until golden on both sides.

Note: These are good alone, with fruit, with maple syrup, or sprinkled with a little powdered sugar and cinnamon. For variety, leave out the banana and blend 2 tablespoons of flour with 1 full cup of the "milk."

Easy Blueberry Muffins

MAKES 8–10 MUFFINS

1 cup whole-wheat flour
1 cup oat flour
1 teaspoon baking powder
1/2 teaspoon baking soda
1 teaspoon ground cinnamon
1/2 teaspoon ground nutmeg
1/3 cup (or less) maple syrup, sugar, or honey
1/2 cup unsweetened applesauce
2 teaspoons vanilla extract
1 cup oat milk
1 cup blueberries, fresh or frozen (if you can find them, wild blueberries are wonderful)

1. Preheat oven to 400 degrees.
2. Mix first six ingredients in a large bowl.
3. Place remaining ingredients in the center. Carefully fold from center to outside until all ingredients are blended. Do not overstir.
4. Spoon batter into a nonstick muffin pan (optional: spray an ordinary muffin pan with nonstick vegetable spray).
5. Bake for 25 minutes, or until tops are brown.

Zucchini Raisin Muffins

MAKES 12 MUFFINS—A GOOD BREAKFAST, DESSERT, OR ANYTIME TREAT

1/4–1/2 cup raisins
1/2 cup oat bran
1/2 cup boiling water
1/2 cup orange juice
1/3 cup honey, maple syrup, or sugar
egg replacer for 2 eggs (2 tablespoons flaxseed meal mixed with 6 tablespoons water, OR 1 tablespoon Ener-G egg replacer mixed with 4 tablespoons water)
2 medium zucchini, shredded (2 cups)
1 cup whole-wheat flour or barley flour
1/2 cup blue or yellow cornmeal
4 teaspoons baking powder
1 teaspoon ground cinnamon

1. Preheat oven to 375 degrees.
2. Put raisins, bran, and boiling water into a small bowl.
3. Stir orange juice, honey, egg replacer, and zucchini together in a large bowl. Add raisin/bran mixture and stir.
4. Stir flour, cornmeal, baking powder, and cinnamon together in a medium bowl.
5. Fold dry ingredients into liquid mixture and stir.
6. Pour batter into a nonstick muffin tin.
7. Bake for 30 minutes, or until a toothpick comes out clean.

The BEST Banana Bread

This is especially good toasted. Use all whole-wheat flour or all barley or spelt flour, if you choose. If you do not have heart disease, add ½ cup chopped walnuts or ¼ cup raisins and ¼ cup walnuts.

1¼ cups whole-wheat flour
1 cup barley or spelt flour
1 teaspoon baking powder
1 teaspoon baking soda
1 teaspoon ground cinnamon
3 small ripe bananas, or 2 large
1 jar baby-food prunes, or ½ cup applesauce
⅓ cup (or less) maple syrup, honey, or sugar
egg replacer for 1 egg (1 tablespoon ground flaxseed meal mixed with 3 tablespoons water OR 1½ teaspoons Ener-G egg replacer mixed with 2 tablespoons water
½ cup raisins
2 teaspoons vanilla extract
¾ cup oat, almond, or nonfat soy milk
1 tablespoon lemon juice

1. Preheat oven to 350 degrees.
2. Mix first five ingredients in a large bowl.
3. Mash bananas in a medium bowl. Mix in remaining ingredients.
4. Add liquids to flour and mix gently. Pour into a 9 × 5-inch loaf pan and bake for 70 minutes, until a toothpick comes out clean.

Safe Cereals

Making breakfast fast, easy, and healthy is no problem these days, given the variety of good cereal choices that are available. Among them:

Oatmeal has limitless possibilities. Make it the usual way, adding water, or try commercial old-fashioned rolled oats uncooked (see the Esselstyn Breakfast, above). Avoid the more processed quick-cooking oats, if possible.

Grape-Nuts are whole grain. **Raisin bran** by Grainfield or Erewhon contains only whole wheat and raisins. **Multigrain flakes** by Grainfield is just whole grains.

Shredded wheat, both the biscuit variety and mini-wheats, contains a single healthy ingredient: whole wheat. But avoid the frosted version, which is loaded with sugar.

Wheatena, made from whole wheat with added wheat germ and bran, offers 5.5 grams of fiber in a 1-cup serving. (Oatmeal, by comparison, has 4.4 grams per cup.)

Uncle Sam, made from whole wheat and flaxseed, is a good source of omega-3 fatty acids, although the whole flaxseed is not easily absorbed.

Ezekiel 4:9 sprouted grain cereal, manufactured by Food for Life, is similar to Grape-Nuts, and comes with or without flaxseed.

You can eat your cereal with your own banana "milk," as seen in the recipe for Barley Oat Pancakes. But here is a chart comparing the contents per serving of other safe milks. It is best to choose the milk substitute that most suits your own needs.

Oat Milk (Pacific)

130 calories 2.5 g fat 110 mg sodium 19 g sugar

Hemp Milk (Living Harvest)

130 calories 3 g fat 120 mg sodium 15 g sugar

Almond Milk (Pacific)

80 calories 2 g fat 80 mg sodium 7 g sugar

Nonfat Soy Milk (Westsoy)

70 calories 0 g fat 105 mg sodium 9 g sugar

Low-fat Soy Milk (Westsoy)

90 calories 1.5 g fat 90 mg sodium 7 g sugar

Soy Dream Original (Imagine Foods)

130 calories 4 g fat 140 mg sodium 9 g sugar

Silk Soy Milk, unsweetened (White Wave)

80 calories 3 g fat 105 mg sodium 1 g sugar

Soy Slender Plain (Hain Celestial)

80 calories 3 g fat 105 mg sodium 1 g sugar

Rice and Soy (EdenBlend)

120 calories 3 g fat 90 mg sodium 8 g sugar

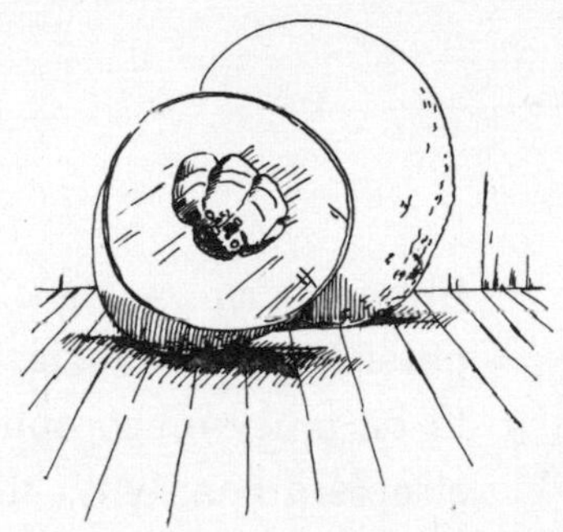

17

Feasting on Salads

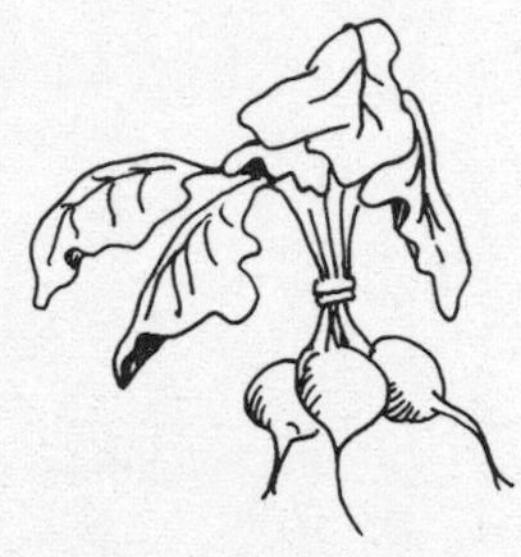

EAT SALAD AT AS MANY MEALS as possible, even breakfast. Salads do not have to be fancy or complicated. They can be simple greens with the dressing of your choice (avoid iceberg lettuce, which is low in nutritional value). Or they can be the main course, brimming with beans, rice, and colored vegetables. In the summer, it is especially easy to make dinner of salad alone. During the tomato season, almost every meal of ours includes thick-sliced tomatoes with basil and balsamic vinegar on top.

Lots of salad suggestions follow. For each recipe, I have provided an estimate of how many servings it makes, but portion sizes are really a matter of individual taste; Essy and I often eat as much salad for one meal as ten people eat at a dinner party! Have fun trying new possibilities, but above all, eat greens and lots of your favorite colored vegetables as often as possible.

Note: A few of these salad recipes include built-in dressings. But please see Chapter 18 for a wide variety of dressing recipes—and for a discussion of no-tahini hummus, a critical ingredient of many dressings.

Bean and Artichoke Salad

MAKES 6 SERVINGS

A pretty salad that tastes as good as it looks. Consider buying artichoke bottoms instead of the tops and cutting each into four strips.

1 large tomato, chopped (2 cups)
1 red bell pepper, seeded and chopped (1/2 cup)
1 small red onion, chopped (1/2cup)
1 cup chopped parsley or cilantro
1 19-ounce can red kidney beans, drained and rinsed
1 15-ounce can chickpeas, drained and rinsed
1 14-ounce can artichoke hearts, drained and rinsed
2 tablespoons fresh lemon juice
2 tablespoons balsamic vinegar
1 1/2 teaspoons spicy brown mustard (or other mustard of your choice)
1 teaspoon dried basil
1 teaspoon dried oregano
1 teaspoon dried thyme
1 garlic clove, minced

1. Combine first seven ingredients in a large bowl.
2. Combine remaining ingredients in a small bowl, stir with a whisk, and pour over bean mixture. Chill before serving.

Quickest Black Bean Salad

MAKES 4 SERVINGS

We could eat this for every meal in summer, even breakfast. It is the salad I make when I have to take a dish to an event, because it is so quick to assemble, everyone comes back for seconds, and it is the best advertisement for delicious NO-OIL eating. It is easy to expand by adding more tomatoes or frozen corn. As always, use LOTS of cilantro.

2 15-ounce cans black beans, drained and rinsed WELL!
1 very large tomato, chopped
1 16-ounce package of frozen corn
½ Vidalia onion, chopped
1 6-ounce can sliced water chestnuts, drained and rinsed
1 bunch cilantro, chopped
½ lime and zest
3 tablespoons balsamic vinegar, or more to taste

1. Put beans, tomato, corn, onion, and water chestnuts in a bowl (glass looks pretty) and mix. Rinsing the beans well keeps the salad from looking gray.
2. Add cilantro, lime, and balsamic vinegar and mix again. Serve alone or with cucumber open-faced sandwiches for a perfect meal.

Black Bean Salad with Balsamic-Lime Dressing

MAKES 4 SERVINGS

1 15-ounce can black beans, drained and well-rinsed
1 large tomato, chopped (2 cups)
2 ears cooked corn, kernels cut off the cob (or half of a 16-ounce package frozen corn, thawed under running water)
1 red bell pepper, seeded and chopped (1/2 cup)
2 ribs celery chopped (1/2 cup)
1 loosely packed cup (or more) chopped cilantro
juice and zest of 1 lime
2–3 tablespoons balsamic vinegar

Combine all ingredients in the order above, stir, and eat!

Black Bean and Citrus Salad

MAKES 6 SERVINGS

This is a light, wet salad, perfect for a hot summer day, but it is just as good in winter, when it brings lovely memories of summer. Mix all ingredients together in a large bowl.

1 large onion, diced (1 cup)
1 red bell pepper, seeded and diced (1 cup)
6 oranges, sectioned, membranes and pith removed (1 1/2 cups)
2 teaspoons orange zest
1/4 cup fresh orange juice, reserved from orange sections
3 tablespoons fresh lime juice

½ teaspoon ground cumin
¼–½ teaspoon Tabasco or other hot sauce
½–1 cup chopped cilantro
2 15-ounce cans black beans, drained and rinsed
arugula or baby spinach

1. Stir-fry onion and pepper in a nonstick saucepan over medium heat until just tender. Add orange juice or water as necessary. Set aside.
2. Place orange sections in a large bowl.
3. Combine orange zest, orange juice, lime juice, cumin, and Tabasco in a bowl.
4. Add onion mixture, cilantro, and beans to orange sections. Add juice mixture and toss to combine. Serve over a bed of arugula or baby spinach.

VARIATION:

Do not cook onion and pepper, add a little balsamic vinegar, and omit the Tabasco.

Colorful Broccoli Salad

MAKES 6 SERVINGS

2 bunches broccoli, florets in small pieces, stems sliced
2 large onions, quartered and separated
1 red bell pepper, seeded and chopped (1 cup)
3 pieces bok choy, chopped in 1-inch sections, including both white and green parts
4 green onions, sliced
¼ cup rice vinegar

2 tablespoons nutritional yeast
1 teaspoon mustard, any kind
juice and zest of 1 lime

1. Steam broccoli until just tender and bright green, remove from heat, and put in a large bowl.
2. While broccoli is steaming, spread onions on a baking sheet and broil until browned on one side, watching carefully. Turn and brown other side. Remove and scrape into bowl with broccoli.
3. Add peppers, bok choy, and green onions to broccoli.
4. Mix vinegar, nutritional yeast, mustard, lime juice, and zest in a small bowl and pour over broccoli. Chill before serving.

Note: This is a pretty salad, and a meal in itself with whole-wheat bread. If you like lots of dressing, double the quantities in Step 4.

Butter Bean and Basil Salad

MAKES 6 SERVINGS

This has always been our son Rip's favorite salad.

3 15-ounce cans butter beans, drained and rinsed
2 garlic cloves, minced
1/2 cup (or more) coarsely chopped basil
1 16-ounce package frozen corn, thawed under running water
1 box grape or cherry tomatoes, halved, or 1 large tomato, chopped
1 small red onion, chopped (1/2 cup)
juice and zest of 1 lemon
1/4 cup balsamic vinegar

Mix all ingredients and pile in center of a platter or bowl. Surround with spinach leaves and other vegetables of your choice, raw or cooked.

Hot-and-Sour Cabbage Salad

MAKES 4 SERVINGS

We belong to a local community-supported agriculture farm and in the summer get wonderful fresh vegetables weekly. This is adapted from one of the CSA recipes.

1/2 head Napa cabbage, shredded
1 green onion, thinly sliced
1/4 cup seasoned or plain rice vinegar
1 tablespoon peeled, minced fresh ginger
1 teaspoon sugar (optional)
1/2–3/4 teaspoon red pepper flakes

1. Place cabbage and green onion in a large bowl.
2. In a small saucepan, over medium heat, bring vinegar, ginger, sugar (optional), and hot pepper flakes to a boil, stirring until sugar dissolves. Pour hot dressing over cabbage and toss.

Easy, Fabulous Corn Salad

MAKES 3–4 SERVINGS

1 16-ounce package frozen corn, thawed under hot water, or 3 ears cooked corn off the cob
1 large red bell pepper, seeded and diced (1 cup)
3–4 green onions, chopped, both white and green parts
cilantro or parsley—lots!
juice and zest of 1–2 limes
balsamic vinegar, to taste
greens

Mix first five ingredients in a bowl. Add vinegar 1 tablespoon at a time until it suits your taste. Serve on a bed of greens.

Roasted Corn and Black Bean Salad

MAKES 4 SERVINGS

This is a wonderful summer salad, and with whole-grain bread, it makes a perfect meal. Add water chestnuts or chopped peppers for variety. If you're in a hurry, don't roast the corn.

2 15-ounce cans black beans, drained and rinsed
1 16-ounce package frozen corn
2 Vidalia onions, thinly sliced and slices halved
3 medium tomatoes, diced (2 cups)
1 bunch cilantro, chopped
6 tablespoons balsamic vinegar
romaine lettuce or arugula

1. Put black beans in a bowl.
2. Spread corn on a baking sheet, broil until just turning brown, and add to beans.
3. Spread sliced onions on a baking sheet and broil until brown and limp. Add onions to beans and corn.
4. Add tomatoes and cilantro to bowl.
5. Add balsamic vinegar, mix well, and serve on a bed of romaine lettuce or arugula.

Gingered Soba Noodles

MAKES 4–5 SERVINGS

1 8-ounce package whole-grain soba noodles
3 tablespoons rice vinegar
2 tablespoons low-sodium tamari or Bragg Liquid Aminos
2 teaspoons peeled, chopped fresh ginger
2 garlic cloves, finely chopped
½–1 jalapeño pepper
2 green onions, chopped
¼–½ cup chopped cilantro

1. Cook soba noodles according to package directions. Rinse and drain well.
2. Mix noodles with remaining ingredients in a large bowl. You might choose to sprinkle a teaspoon of toasted sesame seeds on top. Refrigerate.

Note: The tamari in this recipe makes it high in sodium, but oh, so good!

Lentil Salad, Antonia's Way

MAKES 4 SERVINGS

Antonia Demas, an expert on plant-based nutrition, has a special touch with food.

1 cup uncooked red lentils (2 cups cooked)
1 red onion, diced (1 cup)
1 red bell pepper, diced (½ cup)
½ cup chopped Italian parsley or cilantro
2 tablespoons wine or cider vinegar

2 garlic cloves, crushed
2 tablespoons Dijon mustard
2–3 tablespoons lemon juice
2 tablespoons chopped dill

1. Bring 2 cups of water to a boil. Add uncooked lentils and simmer for 15 minutes, until the lentils are soft but still have their shape.
2. Add chopped onion, pepper, and parsley to warm lentils.
3. Whisk together vinegar, garlic, mustard, lemon juice, and dill in a small bowl. Pour over warm lentil mixture, and mix well.

Note: This salad improves in flavor if it is allowed to marinate. If you overcook the lentils, just proceed. The salad is just as delicious. Leftover lentil salad makes a good filling for sandwiches on whole-grain bread with lettuce and a tomato slice. Red lentils make this salad especially pretty, but they mush quickly. Brown lentils hold their shape better.

Mango-Lime Bean Salad

MAKES 2 SERVINGS

Everyone loves this, so double or even triple the recipe! It vanishes in a flash, and also works well as a salsa. It really is our all-time favorite summer salad. The red onion adds a dash of color. The zest (the peel) intensifies the flavor.

1 mango, peeled and diced
red or Vidalia onion, diced, to taste (start with 1/2 onion)
1 15-ounce can cannellini beans, drained and rinsed
cilantro—1/2 cup or more
juice and zest of 1 juicy lime
baby lettuce or arugula

Combine all ingredients. Serve on a bed of baby lettuce.

Red, Red, Red, Red Salad

MAKES 8 SERVINGS

1 bunch radishes, greens removed, trimmed, and cut into bite-size pieces
½ head red cabbage, cored and chopped
1 box grape tomatoes, halved
2 19-ounce cans red kidney beans, drained and rinsed
1 large red bell pepper, seeded and diced (1 cup)
½ large red onion, diced (1 cup)
2 tablespoons no-tahini hummus
juice and zest of 1 lemon
2 tablespoons balsamic vinegar (or other vinegar of choice)
arugula or baby lettuce

1. Combine first six ingredients in a bowl.
2. Combine next three ingredients in a small bowl.
3. Add dressing to vegetables, toss, and refrigerate.
4. Just before serving, line a shallow salad bowl with arugula or baby lettuce and fill with salad mixture.

Note: This is colorful and filling—and tastes even better if you allow the dressing and vegetable flavors to mix before serving. Double the last three ingredients if you like lots of dressing.

Rice Salad with Apricot-Tamari Dressing

MAKES 8 SERVINGS

2 cups short-grain brown rice (uncooked) or 4 cups cooked
4 cups water

1 carrot, shredded (about 1 cup)
3 ribs celery, diced (3/4 cup)
1 bunch green onions, sliced
1 large red bell pepper, seeded and diced (1 cup)
2 cups corn (fresh off the cob, or 1 16-ounce package frozen, thawed under water)
1 cup frozen peas
1 8-ounce can water chestnuts, sliced

DRESSING:
1/4 cup low-sodium tamari or Bragg Liquid Aminos
3/4 cup rice vinegar
3/4–1 cup pineapple juice
1/4 cup low-sugar apricot jam
2 teaspoons minced garlic
1 teaspoon garlic powder
1 teaspoon onion powder
1 teaspoon dry mustard
2 tablespoons peeled, grated fresh ginger
1 1/2 teaspoons five-spice powder (optional)

1. Cook rice in 4 cups of water for 40 minutes, until all water is absorbed.
2. Assemble all vegetables in a bowl.
3. Whirl all dressing ingredients in a blender until ginger is puréed.
4. Toss vegetables, rice, and dressing together.
5. Serve at room temperature.

Note: If you use tamari, this recipe will be high in salt.

Sweet Potato, Corn, and Green Bean Salad

MAKES 6 SERVINGS

2 medium sweet potatoes, peeled and cut into 1-inch cubes
2 cups green beans, about 1½ inches long
1 cup thawed frozen corn

1. Steam sweet potatoes up to 15 minutes, until tender.
2. Steam green beans 6 minutes, or until tender.
3. Rinse frozen corn under warm water.
4. Put all vegetables in a large bowl. Stir in dressing of your choice (I particularly recommend balsamic dressing; see Chapter 18).

Note: More of any of the ingredients is fine. Use the whole bag of frozen corn or 2 or 3 tomatoes or other vegetables you have on hand. Leftover brown rice is good, as are water chestnuts.

Sweet Potato–Lime Salad

MAKES 4 SERVINGS

I always bake way more yams and sweet potatoes than we actually eat because they are so good cold or in other dishes. Leftover yams and sweet potatoes resulted in this dish.

3 large sweet potatoes and/or yams, cut in bite-size pieces (4 cups)
1 bunch green onions, chopped (about ½ cup)
1 red bell pepper, seeded and chopped (1 cup)
½ sweet onion, chopped
4 ribs celery, chopped (about 1 cup)

2 tablespoons balsamic vinegar
juice and zest of 1–2 limes (about 2 tablespoons of juice, or to taste)
1/2 cup chopped parsley or cilantro

1. Steam sweet potatoes 10–12 minutes, until tender but still firm, or bake at 400 degrees until just tender. Peel and cube. Place in a bowl.
2. Add green onions, red pepper, onions, celery, vinegar, lime juice and zest, and parsley. Mix.

Note: This is a cool and satisfying hot-summer-night salad. If the sweet potatoes get too soft, it tastes just as good. Use both yams and sweet potatoes for a beautiful color combination.

Truly Vegetable Tabouli

MAKES 10 SERVINGS

Bulgur cooks in a flash. It is usually available in bulk—with no added ingredients—in health food stores.

1 cup bulgur
1 cup boiling water
2 large tomatoes, diced (2 1/2–3 cups)
1 cup finely chopped parsley, firmly packed
1 large garlic clove, chopped
4 green onions, white and green parts, chopped
1 small sweet onion, chopped
1 cucumber, peeled and diced
1/4 cup chopped fresh mint
zest of 1–2 lemons
1/2 cup fresh lemon juice
1/4 cup balsamic vinegar
arugula, spinach, or romaine lettuce

1. Rinse bulgur in a strainer, place in a large bowl, and cover with boiling water. Cover and let sit while dicing tomatoes.
2. Drain bulgur well and return to bowl. Add diced tomatoes, mix well with bulgur, and allow bulgur to absorb tomato juice.
3. Add parsley, garlic, green onions, sweet onion, and cucumber to the bulgur mixture.
4. Add lemon zest, juice, and balsamic vinegar and mix well.
5. Refrigerate—overnight if possible, or at least a few hours—and serve on a bed of arugula, spinach, or romaine lettuce.

Note: You can top this, if you wish, with grated carrots, sliced radishes, finely chopped peppers of any color, diced bok choy, or other vegetables. For a heartier salad, add 1 can of rinsed chickpeas and/or thawed frozen corn or cooked kernels cut off the cob.

Mixed Vegetable Salad with Ginger-Orange Dressing

MAKES 8 SERVINGS

2 cups baby carrots
1 whole cauliflower, cut into florets (about 2 cups)
2 cups sugar snap peas
½ cup fresh orange juice
1 teaspoon orange zest
1½ tablespoons lemon juice
2 teaspoons peeled, grated fresh ginger, or more to taste
½ teaspoon freshly ground pepper

1. Place carrots in 2 quarts boiling water and cook about 6 minutes, until tender. Drain and cool under cold water.
2. Repeat with cauliflower florets, cooking for about 4 minutes, until tender.

3. Repeat with sugar snap peas, cooking for 30 seconds, until just tender.
4. Combine remaining ingredients in a small bowl, mix well, and wait to pour over vegetables just before serving.

The Crowes' Vidalia Sweet Mustard Relish Pasta Salad

MAKES 4–6 SERVINGS

After Essy's patient Joe Crowe and his wife, Mary Lind, came to our house for lunch, Mary Lind dropped off a package with a note: "Vidalia Sweet Mustard Relish available in grocery stores is one of our favorite staples. I use it as a dressing in potato salads, rice salads, and pasta salads. Sometimes I use baby corn, artichokes, or hearts of palm just to be exotic." She included a jar of the relish and the following recipe:

½ pound whole-wheat pasta
Vegetables (red, yellow, orange, and/or green peppers, green onions, zuchini, yellow squash, broccoli, tomatoes, cauliflower, etc.)
1 can beans of choice
Vidalia sweet mustard relish, to taste

1. Cook pasta according to package directions. Drain and chill.
2. Cut vegetables into bite-size pieces. Add to pasta.
3. Drain beans. Add to pasta.
4. Add relish to taste. Toss before serving.

Watermelon and Cherry Tomato Perfect Summer Salad

MAKES 6 SERVINGS

This is a most refreshing summer salad. It is good with everything—or by itself as a snack.

2 boxes cherry or grape tomatoes, halved
1 bunch cilantro (2 handfuls), chopped
3 green onions, white and green parts, chopped
½ medium watermelon, cut into bite-size pieces (use a melon baller)
3 tablespoons lemon juice and zest of one lemon
3 tablespoons balsamic or sherry vinegar

1. Put halved tomatoes in a large salad bowl.
2. Sprinkle chopped cilantro and green onions over the tomatoes.
3. Just before serving, add melon balls, lemon juice, zest, and vinegar and mix.

Yam–Yukon Gold Potato Salad

MAKES 10 SERVINGS

5 cups peeled and cubed yams
5 cups cubed Yukon gold potatoes (peeled or unpeeled)
1 12.3-ounce package light silken tofu
¼ cup no-tahini hummus
4 tablespoons balsamic or apple cider vinegar
juice of 1 lime, or more to taste
3 tablespoons nutritional yeast

1 medium red onion, chopped (1/2 cup)
2 garlic cloves, minced
3–4 ribs celery, chopped (3/4–1 cup)
3 tablespoons drained capers
2 teaspoons dried basil, or a handful of fresh basil, chopped
greens or arugula

1. Put yams and potatoes in separate saucepans full of water. Bring each to a boil and cook 5–8 minutes, until just tender. Keep checking. Drain separately and set aside.
2. Combine tofu, hummus, and vinegar in a food processor and process until smooth. Add lime juice and nutritional yeast and process until smooth.
3. Combine potatoes, yams, onion, garlic, and celery in a large bowl. Add tofu mixture, capers, and half of basil. Chill for at least 1 hour. Sprinkle with remaining basil before serving on a bed of greens or arugula.

Note: There are endless potential additions to this salad. Add, according to taste: green onions, red peppers, halved cherry tomatoes, cilantro, parsley, saffron for a nice yellow color, lemon, etc.

Zeb's Rice and Raw Corn Salad

MAKES 6 SERVINGS

Our son Zeb, who lives in California, eats this all the time for dinner. It is good! We were surprised at how good. And it is a meal in itself. The raisins add unexpected sweetness and the toasted sesame seeds add their touch of magic. Try the Orange Juice–Lime Salad Dressing in Chapter 18, or use another salad dressing of your choice.

2 cups cooked brown rice
corn cut off 2 cobs, uncooked

2 medium tomatoes, chopped (about 2 cups)
1 cucumber, peeled, sliced, and halved
¼ cup raisins
4 cups mesclun salad greens
2 tablespoons sesame seeds (optional)

1. Combine all ingredients except sesame seeds in a bowl.
2. Grind sesame seeds, then carefully toast in a nonstick pan or in a toaster oven until just browned. Watch carefully so they don't burn.
3. Toss salad with your choice of dressing, then sprinkle with sesame seeds.

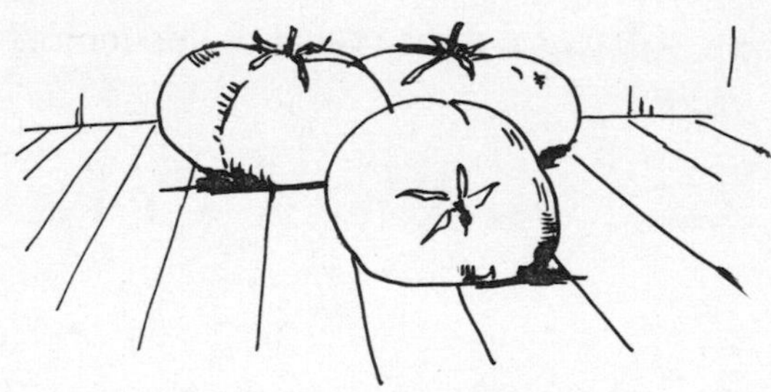

18

Sauces, Dips, Dressings, and Gravies

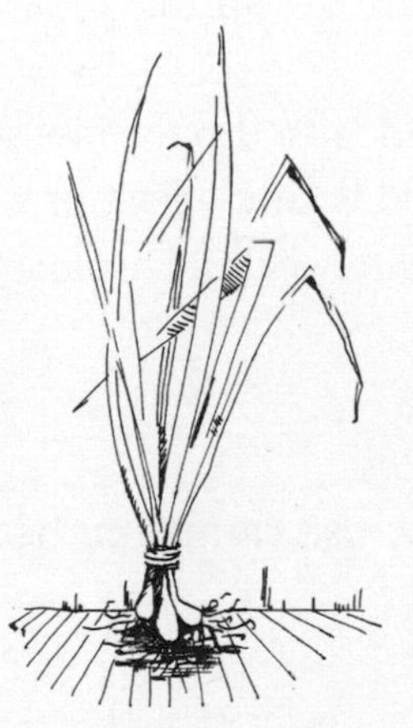

First, a word about hummus. Hummus—*without tahini,* which is high in fat—is the basis for much of what we eat, from a spread for sandwiches or crackers and a dip for vegetables to our favorite salad dressings. We have found two types of commercial hummus without tahini, from Sahara Cuisine and Oasis Mediterranean Cuisine. If those are not available to you, experiment with making your own. Use chickpeas, garlic, and lemon as a base, then try small amounts of other ingredients—peppers, cucumbers, onions, cauliflower, celery, carrots, jalapeño, cilantro, parsley, vinegar, cayenne, spices. When you find the right combination, make big batches to keep on hand. Some suggestions follow.

Simple No-Tahini Hummus

MAKES ABOUT 2 CUPS

1 15-ounce can chickpeas (2 cups cooked), drained and rinsed
2 garlic cloves, chopped
zest of 1 lemon
2–3 tablespoons fresh lemon juice
4 tablespoons vegetable stock or water
1 teaspoon low-sodium tamari or Bragg Liquid Aminos (optional)

1. Combine chickpeas, garlic, lemon zest, lemon juice, and stock in a food processor and process until smooth. Add more stock if too thick.
2. Taste and add as little tamari as possible. (With 3 tablespoons of lemon juice, you probably won't need extra seasoning.)

Note: This is wonderful as a sandwich spread, as a dip for raw vegetables or crackers, as a salad dressing, mixed with vinegar, or with vegetables like Brussels sprouts, broccoli, cauliflower, and asparagus.

VARIATION:

Add 1 cup loosely packed cilantro or parsley; use cannellini beans instead of chickpeas.

Everything Hummus

MAKES ABOUT 3 CUPS

1 15-ounce can chickpeas, drained and rinsed
juice and zest of 1 lemon
3 tablespoons chickpea liquid, vegetable stock, or water

3 baby carrots
2 heaping tablespoons chopped red bell pepper
2 heaping tablespoons chopped onion
1 teaspoon seeded and chopped jalapeño pepper
2 tablespoons chopped celery
3 tablespoons chopped peeled cucumber
1 teaspoon Bragg Liquid Aminos or low-sodium tamari
2 tablespoons cilantro or parsley leaves

Combine all ingredients in a food processor and process until smooth. Perfect on sandwiches, as a dip, or as a salad dressing with added balsamic or regular vinegar. It is even good by the fingerful!

Lori's Hummus

MAKES ABOUT 3 CUPS

Lori Perry, whose husband, Al, is a patient, sent us this recipe.

2 19-ounce cans chickpeas, drained and rinsed
1 12-ounce jar roasted peppers, including liquid
1 teaspoon ready-to-use chopped garlic, or 2 garlic cloves, chopped
1–3 teaspoons lemon juice
1 teaspoon ground cumin

Combine all ingredients in a food processor and process until smooth. Add a little water if the consistency is too thick.

Note: If you find it needs salt, you can add a bit of Bragg Liquid Aminos or low-sodium tamari, but first try using more lemon, which may solve the problem all by itself.

Hummus with Green Onions

MAKES 1 CUP

½ cup plus 2 tablespoons no-tahini hummus
½ cup chopped green onion, white and green parts
2 teaspoons Dijon mustard

Combine all ingredients in a bowl and mix well. This is wonderful stuffed in scooped-out new potatoes or with vegetables and crackers.

Artichoke-Bean Dip

MAKES ABOUT 3 CUPS

1 14-ounce can artichoke hearts in water, drained and rinsed
1 15-ounce can navy or pinto beans, drained
2 tablespoons lemon juice
1 garlic clove, chopped
2 green onions, white and green parts, chopped
pepper, to taste
cayenne, to taste

Combine all ingredients in a food processor and process until smooth. This is good with vegetables, cooked greens, crackers, bread, or just alone.

Best Black Bean Salsa

MAKES ABOUT 4 CUPS

1 16-ounce jar salsa
1 15-ounce can black beans, drained and rinsed
juice of 1/2 juicy lime
cilantro, LOTS!

Mix all ingredients together and put on toasted whole-wheat pita or no-fat, whole-grain crackers. This is also good as a topping on rice. We use it all the time for hors d'oeuvres and find usually none is left!

Special Chutney

MAKES 1 CUP

1 small onion, finely chopped (1/2 cup)
1 small apple, finely chopped (1/2 cup)
1/3–1/2 cup finely diced pineapple
1/4 cup finely chopped red bell pepper
1 tablespoon raisins, soaked in hot water until plumped, drained and finely chopped
1 teaspoon Madras curry powder
1/2 cup rice vinegar
black pepper, to taste

1. Cook onion in a nonstick saucepan 2 minutes, until translucent. Use water as needed.
2. Toss in apple, pineapple, pepper, raisins, and curry powder and cook 1–2 minutes, until fruit is tender but not mushy.

3. Pour in rice vinegar, bring to a boil, and cook until the liquid is reduced by half. The chutney is delicious on brown rice or with curry dishes.

Sweet Corn Sauce

MAKES ABOUT 1½ CUPS

This sauce is adapted from the Casa de Luz Community Cookbook. *It is easy and quick, and looks pretty with parsley, cilantro, or dill sprinkled on top. Use it on greens or grains.*

5 ears uncooked fresh corn (preferred), or 1 16-ounce package frozen corn
1 small onion, chopped (½ cup)
½ cup vegetable broth or water

1. Cut corn off cob and scrape cobs to extract juice. If you are using frozen corn, thaw under running water.
2. Place all ingredients in a blender and process until smooth.
3. Put blended mixture in a pan and cook like scrambled eggs until it thickens. Add water if necessary. A thinner sauce is better over greens. This also makes a good salad dressing just as it is, or add vinegar, lemon, or lime to taste.

Basic White Sauce

MAKES ABOUT 1 CUP

1 tablespoon whole-wheat flour
1 tablespoon cornstarch or arrowroot
1 tablespoon low-sodium tamari
pepper, to taste
½ cup vegetable broth
½ cup oat, almond, or nonfat soy milk

1. Combine first four ingredients in a saucepan.
2. Slowly add vegetable broth and milk, stirring to avoid lumps.
3. Cook over medium high heat, stirring until sauce is smooth and begins to thicken.

VARIATIONS:

For lemon sauce, make basic white sauce and add 2 tablespoons lemon juice plus zest of 1 lemon. For garlicky white sauce, add 1/2 teaspoon garlic powder, 1 tablespoon onion powder, and 2–3 tablespoons chopped chives. For mushroom sauce, make the garlicky white sauce, then add 1 cup sliced, stir-fried mushrooms.

Curry Sauce

MAKES ABOUT 3 CUPS

This sauce is adapted from one of my favorite cookbooks, Fat Free and Delicious, *by Robert Siegel. It is good on broccoli, cauliflower, asparagus, rice, or pasta.*

1 cup cooked brown rice
2 cups water
1/4 cup nutritional yeast
1 tablespoon white miso (optional)
1 teaspoon garlic powder
1–2 teaspoons curry powder, to taste

1. Combine brown rice and water in a food processor and process until smooth. It may take a minute or two.
2. Add remaining ingredients and continue to process until smooth. Pour into a saucepan and heat, stirring constantly until just bubbling.

Pea Guacamole

MAKES ABOUT 2 CUPS

This is delicious by itself, on crackers, with vegetables, with beans and rice, or as a spread on sandwiches. It was excellent with Finn Crisp caraway crackers heated to extra crispy in the toaster.

2 cups frozen peas
1 tablespoon plus 1 teaspoon fresh lemon juice
½ teaspoon minced garlic
cilantro, a handful or more
1 small red onion, minced (¼ cup)
½ cup minced ripe tomato
pepper, to taste
red pepper flakes, to taste

1. Put peas under warm water until softened but still cold. Drain well. Place peas, lemon juice, garlic, and cilantro in a food processor and process until very smooth. Transfer to a medium bowl.
2. Stir in onion, tomato, pepper, and pepper flakes. Let stand for 10 minutes and serve within an hour or two. (If it sits around longer, it loses its bright color—but still tastes good.)

Pineapple Salsa

MAKES 6 CUPS

This is colorful and so fresh tasting. Eat on burritos, potatoes, crackers, curry dishes—almost anything. It is beautiful on top of brown rice and black beans. Add any leftovers to a stir-fry and then add a little brown rice vinegar.

1 pineapple, peeled and sliced into rings ½ inch thick
1 ripe mango, peeled and chopped

1 large tomato, chopped (1 cup)
4 garlic cloves, minced
1–3 jalapeño chilies, seeded and chopped, or to taste
3 tablespoons (or more) chopped cilantro

1. Grill or broil pineapple rings until lightly browned on both sides.
2. Chop pineapple and mix with remaining ingredients. Chill overnight to allow flavors to mix or eat immediately if you can't wait. It's still good.

Sesame-Honey Tamari Sauce

MAKES ABOUT 2 TABLESPOONS

Use sparingly because of the tamari (sodium) and sesame seeds (fat). This is wonderful on green beans.

2 tablespoons sesame seeds
1 teaspoon honey
2 teaspoons low-sodium tamari

1. Toast sesame seeds in the oven or in a pan, watching carefully so they don't burn. Place in a small grinder or food processor and process just until ground.
2. Put sesame seeds in a small bowl and add honey and tamari. Stir until mixed and just crumbly. Add to hot green beans or use with any vegetable. This recipe goes a long way: it is enough for 1½ pounds green beans.

Miraculous Walnut Sauce

Note: This sauce is *not* for those with heart disease unless used very sparingly.

When we visit our son Rip in Austin, Texas, we always eat at the macrobiotic restaurant Casa de Luz because we love the food—especially the walnut sauce on kale. In the past, we had not eaten much kale. We asked the cook for the recipe for the walnut sauce, and we learned two things. First, you must boil kale in lots of water (now that we know that, we love kale even without the sauce!). Second, there are only three ingredients in the sauce: walnuts, garlic, and tamari. When combined, these ingredients are shockingly delicious and totally transformed. Here's how:

1. Put in a blender or food processor a handful of walnuts, a clove or more of garlic (depending on garlic tolerance), and a big sprinkle of low-sodium tamari.
2. Blend, adding as much water as necessary (about 1/2 cup) to make it the right consistency to pour. It can be quite thin, and goes a long way. And it is good on absolutely everything.

Although it is best to make it according to your own taste, here is a possible recipe:

1/2 cup walnuts
1 garlic clove
1–2 tablespoons low-sodium tamari
1/2 cup (or more) water, depending on how thin or thick you want the sauce

Salad Dressings for All Tastes

You should eat lots of huge salads, so it is very important to find salad dressings you really like.

Dressings can be easy. For instance, you can simply add orange juice, lime juice, and balsamic vinegar to greens without even mixing them first; just add what tastes right to you. Or you can make a marvelous light summer salad simply by adding strawberries, raspberries, and sliced oranges—with their juice—to a bed of baby lettuce, then topping it all with raspberry wine vinegar to taste.

There is a wide variety of dressing recipes suggested below. But do experiment with making your own. Look in all the wonderful books available for more suggestions. Before you know it, you will not miss olive oil!

Hummus Salad Dressing

MAKES 1/4 CUP

After many years—sometimes eating salad with no dressing, more often with just balsamic vinegar—we finally found a salad dressing that is one of our favorites. The basic ingredients are hummus (without tahini), balsamic vinegar, and a little mustard. This sticks to lettuce well. If you have no no-tahini hummus, try using equal amounts of nutritional yeast and vinegar. The following recipe is a basic suggestion, which you can vary according to taste by adding lime, lemon, or orange juice, garlic, or ginger.

2 heaping tablespoons no-tahini hummus
2 tablespoons balsamic vinegar or vinegar of choice
1/2 teaspoon mustard of choice

Mix and pour over greens.

Note: If you want a light-colored dressing, use white balsamic vinegar.

Hummus–Orange Juice Dressing

MAKES ABOUT ½ CUP

2–3 heaping tablespoons no-tahini hummus (see first section of this chapter)
2 tablespoons balsamic vinegar
3 tablespoons orange juice
1 teaspoon mustard of choice
½ teaspoon peeled, chopped fresh ginger

Mix and pour over greens.

Rip's Salad Dressing

MAKES ABOUT ½ CUP

Our son Rip created this recipe. After we gave up oils, it was the first dressing that made us really like salad again. The nutritional yeast—available at health food stores—makes the difference.

juice of 1 lemon, lime, or orange
1 teaspoon low-sodium tamari or soy sauce (optional)
1 tablespoon nutritional yeast
1 teaspoon mustard of choice
1–2 tablespoons (or more) balsamic vinegar or any vinegar of choice
mint sauce (a few drops) or a teaspoon of molasses or honey (optional)

Orange Juice–Lime Salad Dressing

MAKES ABOUT 1/2 CUP

This is an easy, light dressing that is good on almost anything.

1/3 cup orange juice
1 teaspoon peeled, chopped fresh ginger
juice and zest of 1 lime
2 tablespoons raspberry balsamic vinegar

Mix all ingredients. (If you cannot find raspberry balsamic vinegar, use regular balsamic or any vinegar of your choice.)

Jane's 3, 2, 1 Salad Dressing

MAKES ABOUT 1/3 CUP

Every time we eat our daughter Jane's salads we ask, "What is this delicious dressing?" It is easy to make and to adjust to personal taste.

3 tablespoons balsamic vinegar
2 tablespoons mustard of choice
1 tablespoon maple syrup

Mix all ingredients in a small bowl and whisk until smooth.

Fat-free Vinaigrette

MAKES ABOUT ½ CUP

This is Jennifer Raymond's recipe from her wonderful book Fat-Free & Easy.

½ cup seasoned rice vinegar
1–2 teaspoons stone-ground or Dijon mustard
1 garlic clove, crushed or pressed

Whisk all ingredients together.

Gravy Recipes

Gravy makes mashed potatoes, lentil loaf, stuffing, and all grains taste delicious. Start by browning onions and garlic—and then get creative.

Brown Gravy

MAKES 2 CUPS

3 tablespoons whole-wheat flour
2 cups water
1 tablespoon Bragg Liquid Aminos or low-sodium tamari
1 teaspoon onion powder
1 teaspoon garlic powder
⅛ teaspoon dried marjoram
¼ teaspoon ground turmeric
1 teaspoon dried parsley flakes

1. Brown flour in a nonstick pan, stirring constantly. Do not burn.

2. Stir in water slowly.
3. Add remaining ingredients and simmer for 15 minutes, stirring constantly.

Easy Mushroom Gravy

MAKES ABOUT 4 CUPS

This is good on mashed potatoes, baked potatoes, rice, millet, polenta, lentil loaf—even just on toast!

1 onion, chopped
2–3 garlic cloves, minced
1 10-ounce box mushrooms, sliced
vegetable broth, wine, or water
2 cups water
2 tablespoons whole-wheat flour
1 tablespoon miso, low-sodium tamari, or Bragg Liquid Aminos
2 tablespoons sherry (optional)
black pepper

1. Stir-fry onion in a heavy saucepan over medium heat, adding broth or water as necessary. Allow onion to brown a little, scrape the pan, add liquid, and let it brown more, but watch carefully so it doesn't burn. Add garlic and sliced mushrooms and continue cooking until mushrooms are soft. Add vegetable broth, wine, or water as necessary to keep from burning.
2. Add 1 cup of water, stir, and continue cooking.
3. Mix whole-wheat flour and miso in the remaining cup of water, stir, then add to the mushrooms and stir again. Add sherry (optional).
4. Continue cooking until gravy thickens. Add pepper to taste. Keep warm over low heat until serving. Add extra miso or low-sodium tamari to taste, but keep in mind that using vegetable broth instead of water intensifies the flavor.

Shiitake Mushroom Gravy

MAKES ABOUT 3 CUPS UNSTRAINED, OR 2¼ CUPS STRAINED

This recipe is adapted from The Taste for Living Cookbook.

1 medium onion, sliced (about 1 cup)
1 cup shiitake mushrooms, stems removed, sliced
3½ cups water
¼ cup low-sodium tamari or Bragg Liquid Aminos
¼ cup plus 1 tablespoon rice flour or whole wheat flour
1 tablespoon chopped fresh thyme, or ¼ teaspoon dried
2 teaspoons chopped fresh sage, or ½ teaspoon dried
1 tablespoon lavender (optional)

1. Place onions and mushrooms in medium saucepan over low heat. Cover and cook for about 10 minutes, until vegetables begin to exude moisture, stirring occasionally.
2. Add water and tamari or Bragg Liquid Aminos and cook for 10 minutes.
3. Add rice flour, stirring with a whisk to eliminate lumps.
4. Simmer 10 minutes, stirring occasionally.
5. Pour gravy through a fine strainer into a clean saucepan to remove mushrooms and onions, or leave it unstrained for a delicious country-style gravy.
6. Add herbs, heat, and serve.

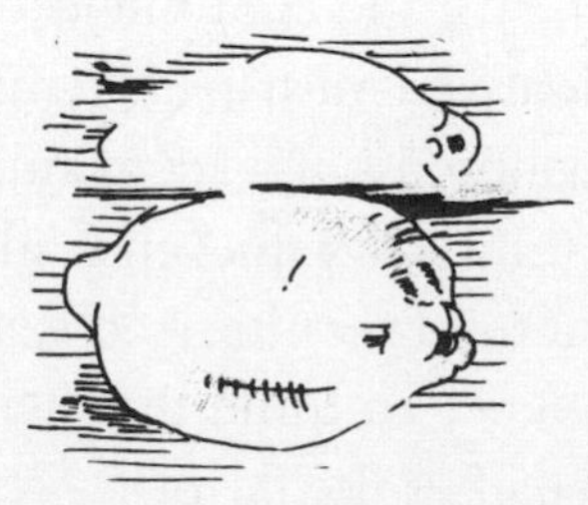

19

Vegetables, Plain and Fancy

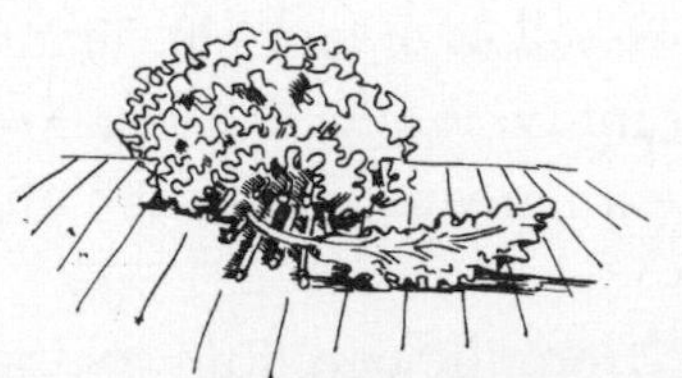

TRY TO STEAM a few vegetables each night with your dinner. Seasonal produce—asparagus in the spring, corn, sliced tomatoes with basil in late summer, and squash in the fall—should fill your plates, along with broccoli, cauliflower, green beans, snap peas, zucchini, Brussels sprouts, and so on. They are all good plain or with lemon juice, a little balsamic or rice vinegar, or salt-free Mrs. Dash seasoning blend sprinkled on top.

Save the water from steaming and use it as a base for soup or as a broth in which you can stir-fry other ingredients. If you have leftover vegetables, toss them into a salad the next day.

It is fun to try new ways to cook old vegetables (see Roasted Cauliflower) or old ways to cook new vegetables (see Beet Greens Surrounded with Beets). And here's a tip: the fast way to "cook" frozen vegetables like peas and corn is simply to thaw them under hot running water.

Beet Greens Surrounded with Beets

MAKES 6 SERVINGS

If you have never eaten fresh beets, you are in for a treat. If you can find pale pink Chioggia beets, they are the best!

2 bunches beets with greens
lemon juice and zest

1. Cut beets off stems (save greens) and put in a large pot of water. Bring water to a boil, then turn to low, and simmer for 30 minutes, or until beets are soft.
2. Wash greens and discard any that are yellow or look old. Tearing by hand or using a knife, cut greens into 2- to 3-inch pieces. Keep some of the stems, if you wish. Steam greens for about 5 minutes, or until done to your taste.
3. Now comes the fun. Remove beets from the pan. Run cold water over them and squeeze off the skins. It's addictive!
4. Slice beets and arrange around the outside of a plate. Sprinkle beet greens with lemon juice and zest in a small bowl in the center.

Children LOVE squeezing the skins off the beets, and it helps make them more willing to try something new. Sweet Corn Sauce or Walnut Sauce, if walnuts are on your diet, are both fabulous on the beet greens (see Chapter 18 for sauce recipes).

Beets with Balsamic Vinegar and Herbs

MAKES 6 SERVINGS

These are wonderful! We first tasted them prepared this way at the 2004 Boston Vegetarian Society meeting and kept sneaking back to the table for more. They will vanish fast, *so make lots.*

2 bunches beets
1½ tablespoons balsamic vinegar, or to taste
¼ red onion, sliced very thin, then chopped into fine pieces
1 tablespoon chopped chives
2 tablespoons chopped parsley

1. Cook beets as directed on page 174, peel, slice, and put into a bowl.
2. Sprinkle balsamic vinegar and onion over beets and mix.
3. Add chives and parsley.

Roasted Beets

Preheat oven to 350 degrees. Wrap one bunch of beets in foil and roast until easily pierced with a fork—about 1 hour for medium beets. Peel and eat.

Note: Roasted beets don't bleed much when cut, so they don't dye everything around them pink!

Broccoli Stir-fried with Orange and Toasted Garlic

MAKES 6 SERVINGS

There is nothing as good or as easy as steamed broccoli with lemon, but for those days when you have time, this is a good change.

1 head broccoli
1/2 cup orange juice
3 tablespoons thinly sliced garlic cloves
1/4 teaspoon red pepper flakes
zest of 1 orange

1. Peel tough skin from stems and cut off florets. Cut stems into one-fourth-inch-thick medallions. There should be about 7 cups of florets.
2. Put 2–4 tablespoons orange juice or water in a wok over medium-low heat. Stir-fry garlic about 5 minutes, stirring frequently, until beginning to brown. Add pepper flakes and stir. Transfer to a small bowl and set aside.
3. Put 1/4 cup orange juice and broccoli in the same wok over high heat, cover and cook, stirring every few minutes until broccoli is tender and orange juice is gone.
4. Stir in garlic mixture and orange zest and eat!

Brussels Sprouts

You will be astounded at how fast they disappear. Our oldest grandchild, Flinn, loved Brussels sprouts so much she took them to her class for her preschool birthday treat. You, too, may become as addicted as Flinn!

Brussels sprouts
no-tahini hummus

1. Trim off base and remove any old leaves, then cut sprouts in half lengthwise. Place in a steamer, cover, and bring to a boil over high heat.
2. Reduce heat to medium-high and steam about 7 to 9 minutes, until tender.
3. Dip sprouts in a no-tahini hummus.

Roasted Cauliflower

MAKES 4 SERVINGS

Our son Rip—a firefighter in Austin, Texas—made this roasted cauliflower for his firehouse and shared the recipe. The first time I made this surprisingly nutty-tasting vegetable treat, Essy and I ate it all!

1 head cauliflower
pepper
Mrs. Dash seasoning blend or herbs of choice
balsamic vinegar
Bragg Liquid Aminos or low-sodium tamari (optional)

1. Preheat oven to 450 degrees.
2. Break cauliflower into florets, and slice to create flat surfaces.

3. Rinse florets and put into a bowl. Sprinkle with pepper and Mrs. Dash seasoning blend or herbs of choice, balsamic vinegar, and Bragg Liquid Aminos, if desired. Mix.
4. Put florets on a baking sheet flat side down and roast for 25–35 minutes, until browned, turning once.

Eggplant-Tomato Melt

MAKES 3–4 SERVINGS

We happened to have an eggplant in our refrigerator one summer day. Essy came home from the store with ten containers of Sahara Cuisine no-tahini Organic Roasted Red Pepper Hummus, and I arrived with a huge basket of tomatoes. Thus this dish was born! The hummus melts like cheese. We had eggplant left over, so dinner the next day was Eggplant-Tomato Melt and lunch the next day was Eggplant-Tomato Melt on toast. We liked it each time again.

1 eggplant, peeled and sliced
garlic granules or powder
onion flakes
1 container no-tahini hummus (buy or make your own, adding *no* tahini)
2 tomatoes, sliced
chopped cilantro or parsley

1. Preheat oven to 450 degrees.
2. Peel eggplant, slice into 1/2- to 3/4-inch pieces, and arrange in a single layer on a baking sheet.
3. Sprinkle garlic and onion flakes on each eggplant slice.
4. Put a heaping teaspoon of no-tahini hummus on each slice. Be generous!
5. Slice tomatoes so that you have as many thickish slices as you have eggplant pieces, trying to match the diameter of the tomato slices to that of the eggplant. Put a slice of tomato on top of the hummus.

6. Bake for 13–15 minutes, or until hummus is bubbling and eggplant is soft. Sprinkle with cilantro or parsley for color, and serve.

Green Beans

MAKES 4 SERVINGS

Trim $1^1/_2$ pounds of green beans. Steam alone or with lemon juice—a staple, for us. Or for a treat, mix Sesame-Honey Tamari Sauce (see Chapter 18) into hot beans. Wow!

Roast Fennel and Apple

MAKES 8 SERVINGS

Before trying this dish, we had not eaten much fennel. We found it surprisingly good.

2 bulbs fennel, cut in $^1/_4$-inch wedges
2 Rome (or any) apples, cut in 1-inch wedges
2 teaspoons honey
$^1/_4$ cup vegetable broth
pepper
low-sodium tamari or Bragg Liquid Aminos

1. Preheat oven to 400 degrees.
2. Toss all ingredients in a big bowl and mix thoroughly. Spread on a baking sheet.
3. Roast 20 minutes, turn over, and continue roasting about 20 minutes longer, until golden and cooked through.

Every-Night Kale

MAKES 4 SERVINGS

Kale is one of the best greens you can eat and is surprisingly delicious just plain, with lemon or vinegar, in soup, or with the sauce of your choice. Try it with Sweet Corn Sauce or, if you don't have heart disease, Walnut Sauce (see Chapter 18 for sauce recipes).

1. Cut off the tough ends from two bunches of kale and remove the spine. Chop into 2-inch pieces and rinse.
2. Put in boiling water and gently cook about 10 minutes, until tender, or to your taste. Superb!

Roasted and Rustic Red Peppers

MAKES 6 SERVINGS

Nothing is as good as these, no matter how you use them. Nothing! I always double the recipe when I make them. If you double the recipe, use the same amount of herbs you would use for six peppers.

6 red bell peppers
3 tablespoons red wine vinegar or balsamic vinegar
2 teaspoons minced garlic
1 teaspoon dried basil
1 teaspoon dried thyme
1 teaspoon dried rosemary
1 teaspoon dried marjoram
1 teaspoon dried oregano

1. Turn the oven to broil. Place peppers on a baking sheet and broil until blackened on one side. Turn and continue broiling until all sides are black.
2. Peel peppers in running water and then slice. Combine peppers with remaining ingredients and marinate for at least 30 minutes.

Note: These are fabulous just plain, on toast, in a sandwich, or in a salad. If you save the juice from the peppers after you roast them, it adds a feel of oil to salad dressings. The easiest way to save the juice is to cool the peppers, then prick them before peeling. Save the juice in the bowl with the peppers themselves.

Festive Squash

Squash is filling, delicious, and easy to prepare. There are many wonderful varieties. Acorn and butternut are good, and if you can find it, Surprise is wonderful. Experiment with different varieties. Delicata, also called sweet potato squash, is especially sweet, and—served with maple syrup—makes an easy and festive holiday dish.

1. Preheat oven to 350 degrees.
2. Cut a delicata or acorn squash in half, remove seeds, and bake for about 45 minutes—inside facing down—in a pan containing about an inch of water. (You can also bake squash whole, then halve and remove seeds after it is cooked.)
3. Remove squash from oven when it is soft. Place cut side up in a pan, drizzle 1 or 2 teaspoons maple syrup in the center of each half, and return to the oven for 5–10 minutes until maple syrup is bubbling and squash begins to brown.

VARIATIONS:

Put a dollop of no-tahini hummus in the hollowed-out squash, then fill with frozen peas, pearl onions, or a combination of peas and onions.

Butternut Squash and Corn

MAKES 6 SERVINGS

This delicious combination is adapted from The Taste for Living Cookbook *by Beth Ginsberg and Mike Milken. Fresh corn is the key. If you have to use frozen corn, however, try Trader Joe's frozen roasted corn.*

1 medium butternut squash
1 15-ounce can corn
4 ears fresh corn, cooked and cut off the cob, or 1 16-ounce package frozen corn
1 teaspoon Mrs. Dash garlic and herb seasoning blend
cilantro or parsley

1. Preheat oven to 350 degrees.
2. Place butternut squash on a baking sheet, pierce several times with a sharp knife, and bake for 1½ hours. Allow to cool at least 30 minutes. (This can be done a day ahead.)
3. Cut squash in half, remove seeds, and put flesh in a blender.
4. Drain and rinse canned corn, place in blender, and puree with squash.
5. Remove to a mixing bowl and stir in fresh corn and Mrs. Dash.
6. Spoon mixture into a casserole dish and cover with a lid or foil.
7. Bake for 30 minutes, until heated through. Garnish with cilantro or parsley. Serve with baked portobello mushrooms, green beans, and salad.

Sweet Potatoes/Yams

Sweet potatoes are delicious baked. Try yams that are orange or sweet potatoes that are pale yellow to see which you prefer. We like a combination. Scrub them well and put on a baking sheet in a 400-degree oven for an hour, or until soft. They are good just plain. Make more than you think you will eat. They are perfect cold, as a snack, or can be used in soup or casseroles.

VARIATIONS:

1. *Sweet Potato Fries.* Slice sweet potatoes, either in thin rounds or French fry–style, and place in a single layer on a baking sheet. Bake in a 400-degree oven for 25 minutes, turn over, and bake another 25 minutes, until the "fries" are as crispy as you want them. Check frequently.
2. *Gingered Yams.* Bake two big yams or three medium ones in a 400-degree oven 1–1½ hours, until soft. Remove skin and mash flesh. Add 1 teaspoon peeled, grated ginger, 1 tablespoon lime juice, and ½ teaspoon curry powder.
3. *Yam, Black Bean, and Mango Delight.* Cut baked yam in half and top with drained, rinsed black beans, chopped fresh mango (the more the better), cilantro, and a little salsa.

Swiss Chard

If you are not familiar with Swiss chard, you have missed a treat! It is spinach-like and delicious, but keeps its volume better than spinach. I try to buy Swiss chard, kale, and beet greens every time I go to the store.

1. Remove stems and tough centers from 2 pounds Swiss chard if desired (they actually taste good). Wash well and cut into thin strips.

2. Put chard in boiling water and blanch about 5 minutes, until just tender. Eat plain, with lemon juice, with Sweet Corn Sauce, or a little Walnut Sauce if walnuts are on your diet (see Chapter 18 for sauce recipes).

Vidalia Onions

You can simply peel these sweet treats, slice them thickly, and spread them on a baking sheet, then roast in a 400-degree oven about 20 minutes, until nicely browned but not burned. They are delicious on pasta or baked potatoes, mixed with other vegetables, in the center of squash or simply eaten plain. Slice fresh garlic and roast with the onions for additional good taste. Or try this variation:

2 Vidalia onions or other sweet onions (Texas Sweets are good), peeled and cut in half crosswise
balsamic vinegar
Bragg Liquid Aminos or low-sodium tamari (optional)

1. Preheat oven to 300 degrees.
2. Put onions in a pan and sprinkle with balsamic vinegar and a little Bragg Liquid Aminos or tamari, if desired.
3. Cover with a lid or foil and bake for a few hours. Even better, if you have enough time, set the oven at 250 degrees and bake all afternoon! You will have a plate of ambrosia for dinner! The longer the onions bake, the sweeter they become. Eat these plain, or serve on brown rice or baked potatoes.

Fried Zucchini

MAKES 2–4 SERVINGS

2 medium zucchini
Bragg Liquid Aminos or low-sodium tamari
garlic powder
onion powder
pepper

1. Cut ends off zucchini and slice lengthwise into at least 4 long slices.
2. Sprinkle a large nonstick pan with a small amount of Bragg Liquid Aminos, then arrange zucchini in pan by wiping each slice, front and back, in the Bragg. Flip the slices around to fit in pan so that each slice will brown.
3. Cook over medium heat for about 5 minutes, then carefully turn over. If pan needs liquid, add a little water or a bit more tamari.
4. Sprinkle cooked side with garlic powder, onion powder, and pepper and continue cooking another 5 minutes, adding tiny bits of water as necessary until both sides are brown. Zucchini this way is so tasty, it is easy to eat lots!

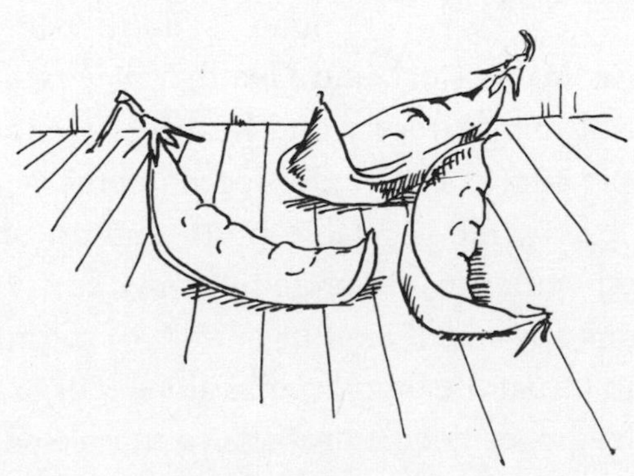

20

Soups, Thick and Delicious

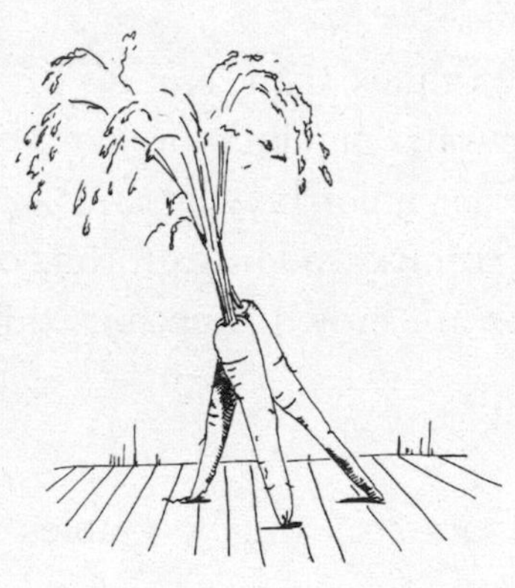

WE LOVE SOUP, especially in cold weather. A good broth makes a difference, and there are some excellent commercial brands to choose from. But I cannot repeat the rule often enough: *Read the ingredients.* Pacific Organic low-sodium vegetable broth, just out on the market, contains only 140 mg of sodium per cup. Kitchen Basics roasted vegetable stock and Health Valley fat-free vegetable broth, available at many grocery and health food stores, have 330 mg of sodium per cup, as has Trader Joe's organic vegetable broth. Pacific makes an organic vegetable broth and an organic mushroom broth, both with 530 mg of sodium per cup. None of these products contains any added oil. But beware of so much sodium.

And you can't trust the brand name alone. For example, Imagine's organic soy ginger noodle broth (440 mg of sodium per cup) and its new organic vegetable stock (580 mg) contain no added oil.

But both Imagine's organic vegetable broth and its no-chicken broth (330 and 450 mg of sodium per cup, respectively) *do* contain added oil, and should be avoided. *Read the ingredients.*

Be wary of the many dry vegetable broth mixes, which are likely to contain added oil and a lot of salt. And most bouillon cubes contain added oil. Seitenbacher instant all-natural gluten-free vegetable broth mix, which is available at health food stores, is delicious and contains no oil, although it is a little high in sodium. And Vegit makes a "very low-sodium all-purpose seasoning."

Best of all, make your own broth. Some options:

1. When cooking beans, add extra water, onions, celery with the tops, carrots, garlic, leeks, and bay leaves. Save the liquid after you drain the beans, then freeze or refrigerate it for later use.

2. Roast onions, carrots, celery, garlic, and leeks at 450 degrees in a heavy roasting pan for an hour. Put roasted vegetables and 8 cups of water in a pot, bring to a boil, then simmer for an hour. Strain off the vegetables and you have a delicious broth that will add flavor to everything from soups to stir-fries.

3. Easiest of all, save the water from steaming vegetables and use it in soups and sauces.

Fill your soup with as many greens as possible. Add the things you like best. If you don't love cilantro, substitute parsley, rosemary, or mint. Boil a little kale and add it at the last minute to keep its color, or add spinach, which wilts quickly, just before serving.

Following are some of the recipes we have enjoyed.

Awesome Almost All-Orange Vegetable Soup

MAKES 8–10 SERVINGS

This soup is wonderfully filling and works as lunch or dinner or even an excellent breakfast, if any is left by then. Serve with whole-wheat bread, and you have a feast!

1 large acorn squash, baked, seeded, and cut in chunks
2 sweet potatoes or yams, baked, peeled, and cut in chunks
1 large onion, chopped (1 cup)
3 carrots, chopped
3 ribs celery, chopped (3/4 cup)
6 garlic cloves, chopped
2 cups red lentils
8 cups water
1 teaspoon dried rosemary
1/4 teaspoon crushed red pepper
3 or 4 handfuls fresh spinach (more if you wish) or chopped kale with the spine removed
3 zucchini, chopped
1 large red bell pepper, chopped (1 cup)
1 bunch cilantro, chopped
3 green onions, chopped

1. Preheat oven to 350 degrees.
2. Bake acorn squash and sweet potatoes for up to 1 hour, until soft.
3. In a large soup pot, over medium high heat, stir-fry onion, carrots, celery, and garlic until onion is soft and carrots are beginning to soften. Add a little water if anything seems to stick. (To save time, skip this step and go straight to Step 4.)

4. Add red lentils, 8 cups of water, rosemary, and crushed red pepper. Increase heat to high and bring to a simmer. Reduce heat to low and simmer 20 minutes, until lentils have almost dissolved.
5. Add acorn squash and sweet potatoes to the pot and mash into the soup. (A potato masher works well.) Cook 10 minutes more.
6. Add spinach and stir into the soup until it wilts. If you use kale, it needs to cook a little longer than spinach.
7. Stir-fry zucchini in a nonstick pan over high heat until just beginning to brown. Add red pepper and stir-fry 1–2 minutes more. (If you are in a hurry, you may omit this step; add uncooked zucchini and red pepper in Step 6.) A few minutes before serving, add stir-fried zucchini and red pepper to the soup mixture.
8. Add cilantro and green onions just before serving.

Beet Soup

MAKES 3–4 SERVINGS

This is another recipe inspired by our CSA (community-supported agriculture). Be sure not to waste the wonderfully nutritious beet greens; steam or stir-fry them and sprinkle with lemon juice or top with Sweet Corn Sauce (see Chapter 18).

1 bunch red beets plus 1 bunch Chioggia or other beets (2 bunches total)
1/2–1 cup orange juice
zest of 1 lemon
2–3 tablespoons lemon juice
mint leaves, to taste (try 6)
pepper, to taste

Boil beets 40 minutes or more, depending on their size, until just tender. Peel. Whirl in food processor with juices, zest, mint, and pepper. Taste, adding more orange or lemon juice, if desired. Chill. Serve with a mint leaf on top.

Note: If you use just Chioggia beets, you'll get a beautiful pink soup.

Best Black Bean Soup

MAKES 7–9 SERVINGS

For three days in a row I made black bean soup, and this is a combination of all three recipes. But it gets its soul from The Moosewood Cookbook.

2 cups dry black beans, or 3 15-ounce cans black beans, rinsed and drained
4 cups water or vegetable broth
1 large onion, chopped (1 cup)
10 medium garlic cloves, chopped
2 teaspoons ground cumin
2 medium carrots, diced
1 cup chopped bok choy
1 large bell pepper, chopped (1 cup)
1½ cups orange juice
2 medium tomatoes, diced (2 cups)
1 large sweet potato, steamed and cubed (1 cup)
black pepper, to taste
cayenne, to taste
green onions, chopped
cilantro, lots!
salsa

1. Soak dry beans overnight or for at least 4 hours in plenty of water. Place soaked beans in a heavy soup pot with 4 cups of water or broth. Bring to a boil, cover, and simmer about 1¼ hours, or until beans are tender. (If using canned beans, skip this step.)
2. In a wok, stir-fry onions, half the garlic, the cumin, and carrots until just tender. Add bok choy, the remaining garlic, and bell pepper. Stir-fry another 10–15 minutes, until everything is very tender.

3. Add vegetable mixture to beans, scraping bowl carefully. Stir in orange juice, diced tomatoes, and sweet potatoes. Add black pepper and cayenne pepper.
4. Puree some or all of soup in batches in a food processor or blender.
5. Simmer over low heat for 10 to 15 minutes. Serve topped with chopped green onions, cilantro, and salsa. The salsa really adds a punch!

Brian's Miso Barley Soup

MAKES 10 SERVINGS

This is another of our son-in-law Brian's recipes. We love it.

6 cups water
1½ cups hulled barley
1 large onion, chopped (1 cup)
2 ribs celery, chopped (½ cup)
8 ounces mushrooms, chopped
2 large red bell peppers, seeded and chopped (2 cups)
2 zucchini, chopped
1 sweet potato, diced and (if you wish) peeled
4 red potatoes, diced
1 bunch collard greens, chopped, with spines removed
2 tablespoons sherry or port (optional)
1 teaspoon garlic powder
4 cups vegetable stock
2–4 tablespoons white miso

1. Bring water to boil in a soup pot. Add barley, reduce heat, and simmer for 1 hour, or until barley is tender. Drain and save barley water.

2. Stir-fry onion in a nonstick saucepan for a few minutes, until it begins to soften. Add celery, mushrooms, and red pepper and stir-fry a few more minutes. Set aside.
3. Steam or boil sweet potatoes and red potatoes until just tender. Drain and set aside.
4. Steam or boil collard greens until soft. Set aside.
5. Combine onion mixture, potatoes, and collard greens with the barley. Add garlic powder and 3 cups of stock and cook over medium heat until soup thickens.
6. Mix miso into 1 cup of warm vegetable stock and stir into soup along with sherry or port, if using. Continue cooking a few more minutes, until soup is warm.

Broccoli Soup

MAKES 6 SERVINGS

2 large onions, chopped (2 cups)
4 garlic cloves, chopped
12 cups broccoli, cut in 2- to 3-inch pieces
4 cups vegetable stock
miso, Bragg Liquid Aminos, or low-sodium tamari to taste (optional)
pepper, to taste

1. Bring onions, garlic, broccoli, and vegetable stock to a boil in a soup pot. Lower heat and cook for 10–15 minutes, until broccoli is tender.
2. Process in batches in a blender until mixture is smooth and brilliantly green, or use an immersion blender right in the soup pot.
3. Add the miso and, if desired, Bragg Liquid Aminos or low-sodium tamari to taste.

VARIATION:

Before serving, add a few handfuls of spinach or chopped red peppers and frozen corn for color, and you have an even more nutrient-dense soup.

Gazpacho

MAKES 4 SERVINGS

Gazpacho, which means "salad soup," is the most refreshing of summer meals. A basic recipe follows, with suggestions for additions, but be creative and add your own favorites.

3 medium tomatoes
1 cucumber, peeled
½ bell pepper, any color, seeded
1 large rib celery
½ large jalapeño pepper, seeded
½ small onion
2 garlic cloves
1 14.5-ounce can no-salt-added diced tomatoes
½ cup chopped parsley or cilantro
2–3 tablespoons balsamic vinegar
juice and zest of 1 lime, at least 1 tablespoon
pepper, to taste
green onions or chives, chopped

1. Chop first four ingredients separately, one by one, in a food processor, pulsing until they are uniformly diced. (You can process the jalapeño, onions, and garlic together.)
2. Combine vegetables in a large bowl. Add diced canned tomatoes, chopped cilantro, vinegar, lime, zest, and pepper and mix. Chill and serve, sprinkled with chopped green onions or chives.

Note: Other ingredients can be added: sliced fresh mushrooms, briefly stir-fried in vegetable broth, wine, or water; 1 can hearts of palm, drained and chopped; stir-fried zucchini, chopped; bok choy, grated carrots, chopped arugula. Use your imagination!

Greek Lentil Soup

MAKES 6 SERVINGS

Connie Collis, the wife of a patient, wrote: "I'm passing on my first recipe that Bill loved, and it is very Greek even without the olive oil and salt." I gave some to our two-year-old granddaughter, and the minute I stopped sharing my bowl with her, she reached for more. This takes thirty minutes from start to finish.

1 16-ounce package brown lentils
6 cups water
2 large onions, chopped, (about 2 cups), or 1 12-ounce package frozen chopped onions
5–6 garlic cloves, chopped
1 14.5-ounce can no-oil tomato sauce
lots of pepper and oregano
3 tablespoons sherry
1 tablespoon brown sugar (optional)

1. Boil lentils in water to cover; drain and rinse. Pay attention to this step or the lentils will not soften.
2. Combine rinsed lentils, 6 cups of water, onions, garlic, tomato sauce, pepper, and oregano in a pot, and bring to a boil.
3. Lower heat to a simmer and cook about 10 minutes, until thickened.
4. Add sherry and brown sugar, if desired, and simmer 20 minutes more.

Antonia Demas' Colorful Lentil Soup

MAKES 6 SERVINGS

1 medium onion, chopped (1/2 cup)
3 garlic cloves
1 green or red bell pepper, chopped (about 1/2 cup)
3 carrots, sliced
2 ribs celery, chopped (1/2 cup)
2 cups tomatoes from a 1 lb. 12 oz. can crushed or diced tomatoes
2 cups lentils, any color
4 cups vegetable broth or water
1/8 teaspoon red pepper flakes
Bragg Liquid Aminos or low-sodium tamari (optional)
1/2 cup chopped Italian parsley or cilantro
baby spinach—lots

1. Stir-fry onion in a large nonstick saucepan until softened, then add garlic, bell pepper, carrots, celery, and tomatoes and stir-fry a few minutes more.
2. Add lentils, broth, red pepper flakes. Bring to a boil. Lower heat and simmer, covered, about 30 minutes, until vegetables are tender.
3. Add cilantro and spinach before serving.

Note: This is good—and colorful, especially if you use red lentils (although other lentils taste just as good). The more greens you add, the more healthful the soup becomes (remember that baby spinach wilts quickly, so don't skimp).

If you have a pressure cooker, brown onions first, then cook on high for 5 minutes. For a delicious main course, serve the lentil soup on top of short-grain brown rice, and surround with steamed spinach.

Marrakesh Express Red Lentil Soup

MAKES 6 SERVINGS

An amazing man who said he's been a practicing vegan for thirty years walked into our son Rip's firehouse in Austin, Texas. He described himself as a retired traveling bum with talents as a cook and a counselor, and he shared the following recipe. He had adapted it from a vegan cookbook, and I have adapted it slightly more. But his words best describe it: "It is a one-pot meal with flavors that are completely transporting. You might imagine lying on embroidered cushions in a Moroccan pavilion, a warm breeze perfumed with spices gently billowing the sheer draperies around you. Bright flowers bloom nearby. You feel warm and relaxed." It makes the kitchen smell wonderful, and it tastes delicious.

1 onion, chopped
4 ribs celery, chopped (1 cup)
water or broth
1 bay leaf
1-2 tablespoons fresh ginger, chopped
½ teaspoon ground cinnamon
½ teaspoon ground turmeric
6 cups vegetable broth
4 plum tomatoes, chopped
1 cup red lentils
1 15-ounce can chickpeas, drained and rinsed
2 tablespoons lemon juice
1 bunch cilantro, chopped

1. Stir-fry onion and celery in water or broth in a large soup pot until tender.
2. Add bay leaf, ginger, cinnamon, turmeric, vegetable broth, tomatoes, lentils, and chickpeas.

3. Bring to a boil, lower heat, and simmer, covered, for 45 minutes, until lentils are tender. Stir occasionally.
4. Right before serving, add cilantro and lemon juice.

Three-Mushroom Barley Soup

MAKES 10–12 SERVINGS

Porcini mushrooms give this soup its delicious flavor. Hulled barley, available in health food stores, is the most nutrient-dense, least-processed barley. It takes about an hour to cook, but if soaked overnight, it cooks faster. Pearled barley, more widely available, is more processed, but still full of nutrients; it cooks in 30–40 minutes.

½ ounce dried porcini mushrooms
1 large yellow onion, chopped (1 cup)
1 carrot, finely chopped
1 rib celery, chopped (¼ cup)
12 ounces fresh mushrooms, thinly sliced
6 medium-large fresh shiitake mushrooms, stems removed, sliced
3 quarts (12 cups) vegetable stock
2 cups hulled barley or pearled barley
1 bay leaf
4 tablespoons balsamic vinegar, or to taste
pepper, to taste
parsley or cilantro
1 bag (3–4 handfuls) spinach

1. Soak porcini mushrooms in warm water for about 30 minutes, until soft. Drain, squeeze out (save liquid to use later in the soup), and chop.
2. Stir-fry onion in a soup pot until beginning to soften. Add carrots, celery, and all the mushrooms. Cook a few minutes, until fresh mushrooms begin to soften.
3. Add vegetable stock, barley, bay leaf, and porcini soaking liquid.

Bring to a boil. Lower heat and simmer for 1 hour, adding more liquid if necessary.

4. Add vinegar and pepper to taste. Before serving, add cilantro/parsley and spinach.

Split Pea Soup

MAKES 8–10 SERVINGS

This is one of my favorites, adapted from The Moosewood Cookbook, *and it's good at breakfast, lunch, or dinner. I happen to love its thickness, but you can make it as thin as you wish simply by adding water. If you eat it right away it is especially colorful.*

3 cups dry split peas
8 cups water
1 bay leaf
1 teaspoon dry mustard
1 large onion, chopped (1 cup)
4–5 medium garlic cloves, crushed
3 ribs celery, freshly chopped (3/4 cup)
3 medium carrots, sliced or diced
5 small potatoes, sliced, then cut like French fries
freshly ground black pepper
3–4 tablespoons red wine vinegar or balsamic vinegar
1 large ripe tomato, diced (1 cup)
lots of chopped cilantro or parsley

1. Place split peas, water, bay leaf, and mustard in a heavy soup pot. Bring to a boil, lower heat, and simmer, partially covered, for about 20 minutes.
2. Add onion, garlic, celery, carrots, and potatoes. Cover and simmer for about 40 minutes, stirring occasionally. Add water if soup seems too thick.

3. Add black pepper and vinegar to taste and serve topped with diced tomatoes and cilantro or parsley—or even better, just mix the tomatoes and cilantro into the soup.

Tip: To make this soup quickly, use a pressure cooker. Brown onions in the cooker, add other ingredients, then turn to high and cook for 8 minutes. For an amazingly delicious variation, combine everything through carrots. Do not add potatoes. Cook until dry peas have completely softened and lost their shape. Transfer some of the soup to a blender and slowly add 16 ounces frozen peas (or use an immersion blender, adding the frozen peas to the pot). Return to pot and heat. Add pepper and more water, if desired.

Spicy Potato Soup

MAKES 8 SERVINGS

There is no need to peel the skins of any potatoes, including sweet potatoes, unless it is your preference.

1 large onion, diced (1 cup)
4 garlic cloves, pressed
2 bay leaves
1 carrot, thinly sliced
2 ribs celery, diced (1/2 cup)
1 large red or yellow bell pepper, seeded and diced (1 cup)
10–12 small to medium red potatoes, cut into 1-inch cubes (or use half sweet potatoes and half red potatoes)
8 cups broth or water
1 teaspoon black pepper
1 teaspoon dried rosemary
1/4–1/2 teaspoon red pepper flakes

spinach or kale, as much as possible
green onions, chopped
cilantro, chopped
Bragg Liquid Aminos or low-sodium tamari (optional)

1. In a soup pot, over high heat, stir-fry onion, garlic, bay leaves, carrots, celery, and pepper in water for 5 minutes. Continue adding water to prevent vegetables from sticking. Cook until all are soft.
2. Add potatoes and water or broth and bring to a boil. Lower heat to low and cook for 30 minutes, or until potatoes are tender.
3. Ladle half of soup mixture into a blender, process until smooth, and return to soup pot (or use an immersion blender right in the pot). Add spices and simmer an additional 15 minutes.
4. Add lots of fresh spinach or kale, and simmer until wilted. (Kale will take a bit longer than spinach to wilt.)
5. Serve topped with chopped green onions and/or cilantro. Add Bragg Liquid Aminos or low-sodium tamari to taste, if necessary.

Pumpkin Lentil Soup

MAKES 8–10 SERVINGS

A great friend sent me this recipe, which we have happily used for years.

1 large onion, chopped (1 cup)
2–6 garlic cloves, diced
3 ribs celery, chopped (3/4 cup)
3 carrots, chopped
2 cups red lentils
7–8 cups vegetable broth or water
1 large can pumpkin (no sugar)
1/4 teaspoon dried marjoram

$^1/_4$ **teaspoon dried thyme**
lots of Tabasco

1. Combine onion, garlic, celery, carrots, lentils, and broth or water in a soup pot. Bring to a boil.
2. Lower heat and simmer, covered, 30 minutes, or until vegetables are soft and lentils have turned to mush.
3. Add pumpkin and spices and simmer until all is blended.
4. Add Tabasco to taste. The Tabasco makes the difference. You will be surprised at how many shakes you need—15 to 20! Be fearless!

Safe Soup

MAKES 2 GALLONS

Richard Klein, a resident who worked with Essy, made this soup after hearing so much about "safe" food. It is one of Essy's favorite soups.

1 16-ounce package frozen mixed vegetables
1 16-ounce package frozen chopped okra
1 16-ounce package lima beans
1 very large onion, cut up, chopped
12 ounces fresh kale, stems removed and chopped
4 large potatoes, chopped
1 pound fresh mushrooms, sliced
1 quart water
1 28-ounce can crushed tomatoes
1 28-ounce can no-oil tomato sauce
2 16-ounce cans whole tomatoes, sliced

THE FOLLOWING ALL TO TASTE:
oregano
black pepper
red pepper

marjoram
garlic powder
whole bay leaves
basil
thyme
cinnamon

Combine all ingredients in a soup pot. Bring to a boil. Lower heat and simmer, covered, for 2 hours. Eat every day for the next week.

Sweet Potato and Lentil Soup with Shiitake Mushrooms

MAKES 4–6 SERVINGS—MAYBE!

This soup is so good that Essy and I ate every bit the first time I made it. If people are hesitant about plant-based food, this could change their attitude!

1 leek, thinly sliced, white part only
6 garlic cloves, minced
2 cups (about 3.5 ounces) fresh or dried shiitake mushrooms, sliced (soak dried shiitakes in warm water for 30 minutes before slicing)
4 cups vegetable broth
2 cups water
1½ cups lentils
1 large sweet potato, scrubbed and diced (it is fine to use the skin)
1 bay leaf
¼ cup fresh basil
pepper, to taste

1. In a large soup pot, stir-fry leek, garlic, and mushrooms for 3–4 minutes, until leeks are soft.
2. Stir in broth, water, lentils, sweet potato, and bay leaf. Bring to a boil.

3. Lower heat, then simmer, uncovered, 30–40 minutes, until lentils and sweet potatoes are soft.
4. Remove bay leaf and puree 2 cups of soup until smooth (or use an immersion blender); return to pot and stir in basil and pepper to taste.
5. Serve as is or over rice with a salad.

Note: This soup is thick. Add liquid to your taste. If you don't have leeks, use onions. The more basil the better. Be daring!

Tomato Soup with Basil and Vegetables

MAKES 6 SERVINGS

1 large onion, chopped (1 cup)
5 garlic cloves, chopped
1 cup fresh basil, packed down
8 ounces mushrooms, sliced (optional)
2 28-ounce cans diced tomatoes (use the lowest-sodium brand you can find)
1/2 cup water
1 1/2 cups tomato juice (K.W. Knudsen organic or low-sodium V8)
pepper, to taste
frozen corn and fresh spinach (optional additions)

1. Place all ingredients except pepper, corn, and spinach in a soup pot and bring to a boil.
2. Lower heat, cover, and simmer for 1 1/2 hours.
3. Just at the end, add pepper to taste and stir in frozen corn and fresh spinach in any amounts you like. If you add all the vegetables, you have a wonderfully healthy soup—or a delicious topping for rice or pasta.

Vichyssoise

MAKES 6 SERVINGS

3 cups cubed potatoes
3 leeks or onions, chopped (2 cups)
2 cups vegetable broth
$^1/_4$ cup (or more) loosely packed fresh basil
pepper, to taste
1 cup oat, or nonfat soy milk
chopped chives or green onions

1. In a soup pot, bring potatoes, leeks, vegetable broth, and basil to a boil. Lower heat, cover, and simmer 20 minutes, until potatoes and leeks are tender.
2. Process mixture in a blender until smooth (or use an immersion blender). Pour into a bowl and stir in milk of your choice. Serve hot, or cover and chill. Top with chives or green onions just before serving.

Wild Rice Vegetable Soup

The hostess of my book group made this soup especially for me. I liked it so much I asked for the recipe. I made the soup for dinner that very night with a number of changes, and we have been enjoying it ever since. It is VERY easy to make, and with the addition of cilantro and spinach has those vital greens!

MAKES 6 SERVINGS

1 cup uncooked wild rice
1 onion, chopped
3 ribs celery, chopped

3 carrots, chopped (2 cups matchstick)
8 ounces mushrooms, sliced
4 cups vegetable broth
2 cups water
1½ tablespoons cornstarch
1 tablespoon vegetarian Worcestershire sauce
hot pepper sauce
pepper
cilantro or parsley, lots
spinach, at least a few handfuls

1. In a soup pot, stir-fry onions, celery, carrots, mushrooms, and wild rice until everything gets just soft.
2. Stir in broth and water. Heat to boiling, stirring regularly. Then reduce heat to low, cover, and simmer 40 minutes until rice is popped and tender.
3. In a small cup, dilute cornstarch with a little water until it is a smooth paste; then stir it into the soup. Cook a few more minutes, until soup thickens.
4. Stir in Worcestershire and hot pepper sauce and pepper to taste and cook a few more minutes. (If using Tobasco start with 10 quick shakes.)
5. Just before serving, add cilantro or parsley and spinach so you are sure to get as many greens as possible.

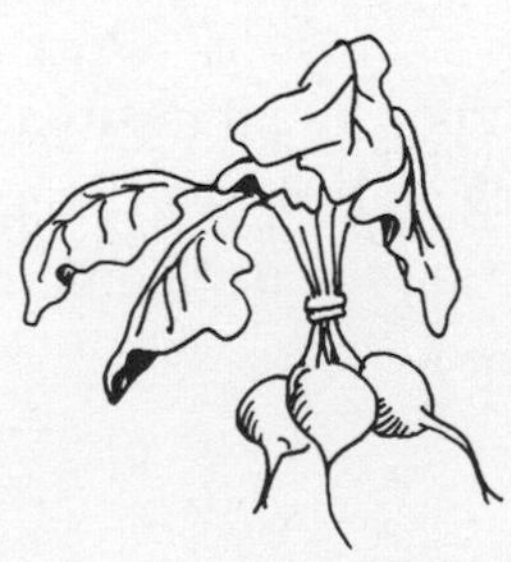

Zucchini-Spinach Soup

Our daughter-in-law Anne Bingham first introduced us to this wonderful, very green soup.

MAKES 4–6 SERVINGS

9 medium zucchini (about 3 pounds)—or really as much as you wish, chunked
1 large onion, coarsely chopped (1 cup)
3 large garlic cloves, chopped
3 cups vegetable broth, or water, or a combination of wine and broth, or a mix of wine and water
2 tablespoons miso, Bragg Liquid Aminos, or low-sodium tamari (optional)
8 ounces (or more, if you like) fresh spinach, coarsely chopped, or 1 box or bag of frozen spinach
2 cups frozen corn
pepper, to taste

1. Combine zucchini, onion, garlic, and 3 cups of liquid in a soup pot.
2. Bring to a boil, lower heat, cover, and simmer about 10 minutes, until zucchini is tender.
3. Place soup mixture, part at a time, in a blender and process until smooth and a beautiful rich green color, or use an immersion blender.
4. Transfer mixture to a pot, and if desired, add miso.
5. Add corn and spinach and any other vegetables you wish. Heat until corn and spinach are warm. (Slightly crunchy spinach is good, so don't cook too long.)
6. Add pepper to taste.

21

Sandwiches for All Occasions

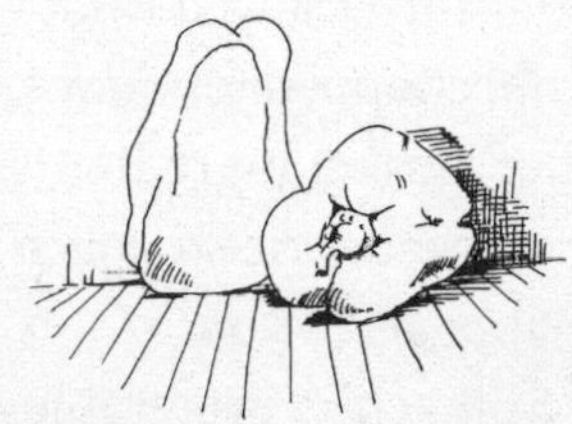

WHEN WE FIRST STARTED EATING a plant-based diet, we had a hard time finding a good substitute for mayonnaise. Then we discovered hummus without tahini, and sandwiches once again seemed as delicious as ever, if not even better. We also like mustard, and a firm called Hudson Valley Homestead makes mustards that are almost like mayonnaise (for information on how to find such products, see Appendix II). There are many mustards with no oil; look for them.

Be very cautious about veggie burgers. Almost all brands contain oil. We have found one safe product: the organic vegan veggie burger from Whole Foods.

For years, Essy's lunch was whole-wheat pita bread filled with leftovers from dinner the night before. It was always fun to see what might end up inside that pita bread! You, too, can make your own miracles with ingredients you love. Toasting bread—wonderful whole-grain bread—always makes a difference.

The Perfect Wrap

This is our favorite way to eat a totally satisfying lunch, and as Essy proudly says, "It is very nutrient dense"—something we strive to achieve in all our meals.

1. Preheat oven to 450 degrees.
2. Assemble nonfat whole-wheat or whole-grain tortillas or flat bread. (Ezekiel 4:9 sprouted grain tortillas work well, and are available in the frozen-food section of most health food stores and many supermarkets.)
3. Spread the wrap with lots of no-tahini hummus. (We have found two commercial varieties, made by Sahara Cuisine and Oasis Mediterranean Cuisine, or you can make your own: see Chapter 18.)
4. Add chopped cilantro, chopped green onions, matchstick carrots (which you can buy in packages), frozen corn thawed under running water or cooked corn cut off the cob, chopped tomatoes, and chopped peppers. You might have other perfect ingredients on hand, as well, such as sliced cucumbers, beans, rice, cooked broccoli, and mushrooms. Add whatever appeals to you.
5. Top with lots of fresh spinach or lettuce. Spinach is preferable, because it wilts better in the oven.
6. Carefully roll the wrap into a sausage-like shape, squishing it together as you go. Cut in half, put on a baking sheet, and bake in a 450-degree oven about 10 minutes, until crisp (keep checking so that it does not burn). Fabulous!

Open-faced Cucumber Sandwich

Mestemacher makes delicious pumpernickel and rye breads, widely available at health food stores, which are good for open-faced sandwiches. But any whole-grain bread will do.

1. Toast whole-grain bread, and spread with lots of no-tahini hummus.
2. Sprinkle chopped green onions on hummus, and top with chopped cilantro.
3. Cover cilantro with a layer of peeled cucumber slices, slightly overlapping.
4. Sprinkle on a little pepper, paprika, or other seasoning of your choice.

Open-faced Cucumber and Roasted Red Pepper Sandwich

This is a little messy to eat but worth the drips! Roasted red pepper all by itself is also good.

1. Toast whole-grain bread, and spread with lots of no-tahini hummus.
2. Cover hummus with a layer of peeled cucumber slices, slightly overlapping.
3. Sprinkle chopped parsley or cilantro over sliced cucumbers.
4. Top with roasted red peppers (see Roasted and Rustic Red Peppers, Chapter 19).

Open-faced Thickly Sliced Tomato Sandwich

1. Toast whole-grain bread, and spread with lots of no-tahini hummus.
2. Top with *thick* slices of fresh tomatoes.
3. Top with lots of fresh basil.

Arugula, Tomato, and Green Onion Sandwich

1. Toast 2 pieces of whole-grain bread, and spread each piece with lots of no-tahini hummus.
2. On bottom slice, top hummus with green onions cut in small pieces, or thinly sliced red or sweet onion.
3. Cover onion with sliced tomatoes. Add arugula or any other lettuce of your choice.
4. Add top slice of toasted bread and press down, so that it all holds together.

Roasted Red Pepper, Cilantro, and Spinach Sandwich

1. Toast 2 slices of whole-grain bread, and spread each with lots of no-tahini hummus.
2. On bottom slice, top hummus with chopped cilantro.
3. Arrange roasted red peppers on top of cilantro (see Roasted and Rustic Red Peppers, Chapter 19).
4. Press a handful of spinach on top of peppers.
5. Add top slice of toasted bread, press down, and slice.

Barbecued Portobello Mushroom, Spinach, and Roasted Red Pepper Sandwich

Our son Zeb was one of the people whose bags got randomly inspected as he was boarding a flight to California. The inspector was fascinated with his sandwiches, and could not get over how healthy and good they looked.

1. Toast a whole-grain bun or bread, and spread no-tahini hummus on one side.
2. Add chopped cilantro, 3–4 strips roasted red peppers (see Roasted and Rustic Red Peppers, Chapter 19), and a grilled portobello mushroom.
3. Top with a stack of fresh spinach or lettuce. Add lid of bun and press down so that it will fit in your mouth!

Better-than-Grilled Cheese

MAKES 4–6 SANDWICHES, DEPENDING ON BREAD SIZE

Although it does not taste like cheese, this recipe, adapted from Breaking the Food Seduction *by Neal Barnard, certainly looks like cheese—and becomes nearly as addictive!*

2/3 cup water
1/4 cup nutritional yeast flakes
2 tablespoons whole-grain flour
2 tablespoons fresh lemon juice
2 tablespoons no-tahini hummus
1 1/2 tablespoons ketchup or tomato sauce
2 teaspoons cornstarch

1 teaspoon onion powder
1/4 teaspoon (or more) garlic powder
1/4 teaspoon ground turmeric
1/4 teaspoon dry mustard, or 1 teaspoon any regular mustard
8 slices whole-grain bread

1. Combine all ingredients except bread in a medium saucepan, and whisk until mixture is smooth.
2. Bring to a boil, stirring with a wire whisk. Lower heat and simmer, stirring constantly, until mixture is very thick and smooth. Remove from heat.
3. Put bread on a grill or nonstick pan, and cover 4 slices with the "cheese" mixture, a thinly sliced tomato, a pile of chopped cilantro, and a few matchstick carrots. Add top slice of bread and cook a few minutes until bottom side of bread is browned.
4. Carefully flip and brown other side. (You may toast the bread before putting on the "cheese" mixture if you want to save time.) These sandwiches squish easily, so be careful cutting them in half. They are so good, it is tempting to eat them every day for lunch or dinner!

Black Bean–Oatmeal Burgers

MAKES 6–10 BURGERS

Betsy Brown, whose husband, Gene, is a patient, created these burgers. She wrote: "I've been thinking about a veggie burger that does not squish. I've decided the first ingredient would have to be concrete." These delicious burgers do squish just a little, but they melt in your mouth.

1 15-ounce can black beans, drained and rinsed
1 14.5-ounce can tomatoes with zesty mild chilies
1 garlic clove, minced, or 1 teaspoon garlic powder

1 teaspoon onion powder
2 green onions, chopped
1 cup chopped carrots
1 cup cilantro or parsley
2 cups old-fashioned rolled oats

1. Preheat oven to 400 degrees.
2. Process first seven ingredients in a food processor until blended.
3. Add to oats and stir.
4. Form into patties, put on a baking sheet, and bake for 8 minutes.
5. Turn oven up and broil about 2 more minutes, until tops are nicely browned. (You can also "fry" the burgers in a nonstick pan until both sides are browned—or grill on the barbecue.)
6. Serve on whole-grain burger buns (the Ezekiel 4:9 brand is especially good) with lettuce, tomato, onion, mustard, ketchup, or no-tahini hummus.

Note: For variety, bake using a favorite barbecue sauce. Heat leftovers in the microwave and eat with a bun or bread, or plain with salsa.

Ginger-Lime Seitan in Sprouted Hamburger Bun

MAKES 4 SERVINGS

Seitan is made from wheat gluten and looks startlingly like strips of beef. Be sure you find seitan that has no added oil.

8 ounces seitan
Ginger Lime marinade & cooking sauce, made by Ginger People, or any barbecue sauce

4 sprouted hamburger buns, no oil added (Alvarado Street Bakery and Food for Life [Ezekiel 4:9] both make good ones), or 8 slices whole-grain bread
4 tomato slices
4 thin slices Vidalia onion
lettuce or spinach

1. Drain seitan, put in a bowl, and barely cover with marinade or barbecue sauce. Let stand for a few minutes.
2. Put seitan and marinade in a nonstick pan and gently stir-fry until lightly browned and warm. Watch closely. Add water if it sticks too much.
3. Put seitan on one side of bun. Top with tomato, onion, and lettuce or spinach, then squish it all down with the top bun. (If you wish, use mustard or hummus, but the seitan is *very* tasty by itself.)

Pita Pizza with Roasted Red Peppers and Mushrooms

MAKES 4 SERVINGS

Nutritional yeast, available at health food stores, looks like cheese but does not change the taste of this delicious pizza.

4 large whole-wheat or spelt pitas
1 large onion, sliced and slices halved
vegetable broth, water, or wine
1 10-ounce box mushrooms, sliced
2 cups pasta sauce, no oil
3 roasted red peppers, cut in small strips (see Roasted and Rustic Red Peppers, Chapter 19)
nutritional yeast

YOU ALSO MAY ADD ANY OR ALL OF THE FOLLOWING:
corn, frozen or off the cob
broccoli, chopped and steamed lightly
artichoke hearts, sliced
tomatoes, chopped
pineapple, chunked

1. Cut pitas in half with a serrated knife. Bake in a 350-degree oven for 3–5 minutes, until edges are lightly crisp. (**Note:** If pita gets hard and looks overcooked, it *still* will be good—maybe even better!)
2. Stir-fry onion in a wok. Add broth, water, or wine, as necessary, then remove onion to a separate dish.
3. Add mushrooms to the wok and stir-fry until soft, adding liquid if necessary.
4. Spread pita generously with pasta sauce, then add onions, mushrooms, and peppers, dividing evenly.
5. Sprinkle with nutritional yeast and bake until pita is crisp and vegetables are warm. Watch carefully.

Note: For a zippier sauce, mix a few tablespoons salsa with pasta sauce. And for an alternate pizza crust, try Nature's Hilights brown rice pizza crust, usually available in the frozen-food section of health food stores (or see Natural Market Place in Appendix II). Follow the cooking directions, then pile high with your choice of toppings.

Roasted Vegetable and Spinach Polenta Pizza

MAKES 4–6 SERVINGS

Our son-in-law, Brian Hart, made polenta pizza for Christmas Day. What follows, a slight variation on the original, is surprisingly filling and really fun to make, as well as beautiful to look at.

POLENTA:

3⅓ cups water
1 cup cornmeal
1 teaspoon garlic powder
1 teaspoon dried oregano
1 teaspoon dried basil

TOPPING:

1 red bell pepper
1 large onion, sliced and slices halved
2 portobello mushrooms, sliced
1½ cups broccoli florets, chopped in 1-inch pieces
1 16-ounce package frozen chopped spinach, thawed
4 garlic cloves, chopped
2 cups no-oil pasta sauce
1 cup chunked fresh pineapple

1. Preheat oven to 400 degrees.
2. Place 3 cups of water in a medium saucepan and bring to a boil.
3. Combine cornmeal with remaining ⅓ cup of water in a small bowl and mix until just barely blended. Spoon the cornmeal mixture into the boiling water and whisk until smooth.
4. Turn heat to low and simmer for about 15 minutes, until very thick, stirring often.

5. Stir in garlic powder, oregano, and basil, then place on a pizza stone or baking sheet and pat into a pizza shape, creating an edge with a flat spatula or with your fingers, as the polenta cools and gets less sticky. Make the polenta as thin or thick as desired, then bake for 15 minutes. (Any leftover polenta is good sliced thinly and "fried" in a nonstick pan.)
6. Put whole pepper, sliced onion, and portobello mushrooms on a baking sheet and broil on top shelf in the oven. Keep turning pepper. The mushrooms will be cooked first. Remove them to a small dish. Turn onions and cook a little longer. Remove when brown to another small dish and keep turning pepper until all sides are black.
7. Remove blackened pepper, hold under running water, remove seeds, peel off skin, and slice into strips.
8. Steam broccoli lightly and drain.
9. Thaw spinach under running water in a strainer. Stir-fry garlic in a nonstick pan with veggie broth, wine, or water, then add spinach and continue stir-frying until liquid has evaporated.
10. Now comes the fun! Spread spinach over polenta. On top of spinach, spread pasta sauce, then arrange portobello strips, onions, broccoli florets, pineapple, and, finally, roasted red pepper strips.
11. Bake for 25–30 minutes.

VARIATIONS:

Substitute any other mushrooms for portobellos; if you don't have heart disease, sprinkle walnuts on the polenta. Or just be crazily creative!

Toasted Garlic Buns

MAKES $^1/_2$–$^3/_4$ CUP, ABOUT 6 SERVINGS

For that great garlic bread taste, try these easy recipes on Ezekiel 4:9 sprouted grain burger buns (see Food for Life in Appendix II, Resources) or any whole-grain bread. It is fabulous with soup or a salad.

4 large elephant garlic cloves, or 2 whole heads garlic
4–6 tablespoons vegetable broth
2 tablespoons chopped parsley or cilantro

1. Preheat oven to 400 degrees.
2. Cut top off elephant garlic and peel off outside skin. Wrap garlic in parchment paper, sprinkle with 2 tablespoons of broth, tightly seal with foil, and roast for 45 minutes. Cool slightly.
3. Mash garlic in a small bowl. Slowly mix in vegetable broth and chopped parsley until mixture has the consistency of softened butter.
4. Spread on toasted buns or whole-grain bread. Even better, toast whole-grain bread lightly, spread with garlic mixture, and re-toast!

If you are in a hurry, here is another *very* garlicky option:

1. Using a garlic press, squeeze garlic cloves into a small dish.
2. Add enough vinegar (any variety), lemon, lime, or other fruit juice or vegetable broth to mix garlic into a paste.
3. Spread garlic on a bun and toast under a broiler until tops are nicely browned.

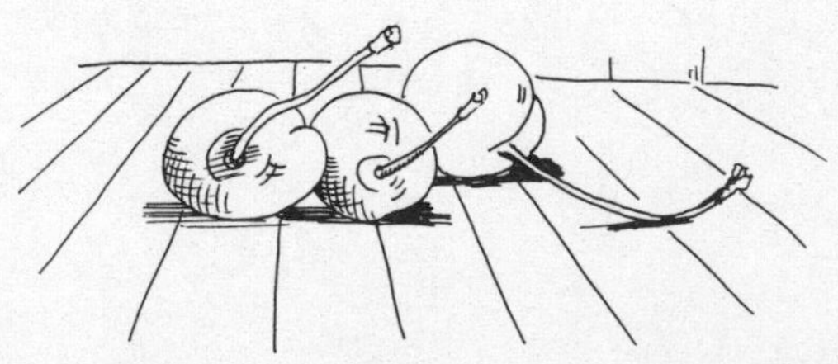

22

The Main Course

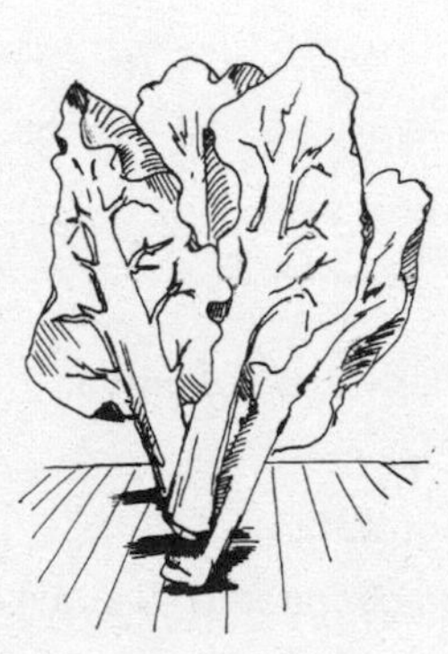

ANYTHING YOU LOVE can be your main course. There are many suggestions here, as well as in Chapter 19 (Vegetables, Plain and Fancy). Create your own version of favorites.

Black Beans and Rice

MAKES 6 SERVINGS

This was our first and favorite nonfat meal, great for guests. Below, you'll find suggestions for vegetables to add to the dish, but be creative. Use what you love!

A note on rice: always use brown rice. It is the most nutritious (just the hull has been removed), and it comes in many varieties. Long-grain rice is light and fluffy. Medium-grain rice is stickier, but fluffier and less chewy than short-grain, our favorite. Basmati brown rice is aromatic. Some of the many others: Chinese black rice, Wehani rice, Texmati rice, and Bhutanese red rice. Experiment until you find your favorites. And don't forget about wild rice. Generally, use 2 cups of water to cook 1 cup of rice, which serves two to four.

There are many ways to prepare the beans. They are delicious warmed straight from the can—liquid and all. If you want less sodium, drain and rinse the beans first, then heat them in water.

2 cups brown rice, uncooked
3 15-ounce cans black beans
2–3 tomatoes, chopped (2–3 cups)
1 Vidalia onion, 1 bunch green onions, or any other variety of onion, chopped
1 16-ounce package frozen corn, thawed under hot water
1–2 red, yellow, or green bell peppers, seeded and chopped (1–2 cups)
1 cup grated or matchstick carrots
1 8-ounce can water chestnuts
1 bunch cilantro, chopped
1 bunch arugula, chopped
low-sodium tamari or Bragg Liquid Aminos
salsa

1. Cook brown rice following package directions.
2. Heat beans either in their liquid or, drained and rinsed, in a little water.

3. Put all chopped vegetables in individual dishes.
4. To serve, start with a base of rice, add beans, and pile your plate high with veggies. Top it all with salsa or a sprinkle of low-sodium tamari or Bragg Liquid Aminos. If you have leftovers, use them for salad the next day, adding balsamic vinegar. Or use the leftovers in a sandwich or wrap with a no-tahini hummus, a slice of tomato, and lettuce. Heaven!

Our family has developed some interesting variations on the basic theme.

Here's the recipe from our son Ted:

For every can of black beans, add 1 teaspoon ground cumin, 1/2 teaspoon ground cinnamon, a handful of raisins, and 2 tablespoons orange-juice concentrate. Just stir these ingredients into the beans in their liquid.

Here's the version from our son-in-law, Brian Hart:

Drain and rinse 3 15-ounce cans of beans. In a nonstick pan, stir-fry 1 chopped onion in 1 tablespoon ground cumin, 1 tablespoon chili powder, 1 teaspoon garlic powder, and orange juice or water as needed for liquid, until onions are soft. Add 1/2 jar of any salsa, juice of 1/2 lime, and 2 tablespoons barbecue sauce (optional) and simmer.

Brazilian Black Beans

MAKES 6 SERVINGS

This is very quick and soooo *good!*

1 large onion, chopped
vegetable broth, water, juice, or wine
2–4 garlic cloves, minced
1 tablespoon peeled, grated, or minced ginger
2 15-ounce cans black beans, drained and rinsed
2 14.5-ounce cans diced tomatoes

1/8–1/2 teaspoon crushed red pepper flakes
cilantro or parsley

1. In a nonstick pan, stir-fry onion in a small amount of vegetable broth, water, juice, or wine until translucent. Add garlic and ginger and stir-fry a few minutes more.
2. Add beans, tomatoes, and pepper. Simmer, stirring, 5–10 minutes, until heated. For a quick and colorful meal, serve over brown rice surrounded by frozen peas, rinsed in hot water. Or instead of peas, try kale with Sweet Corn Sauce (see Chapter 18). Just before serving, add cilantro.

VARIATION:

Add corn, chopped bok choy, or other vegetables of your choice.

Speedy International Stew

MAKES 4–6 SERVINGS

This recipe comes from Betsy, whose husband, Gene, a patient, insisted she send the recipe he loves.

1 15-ounce can black beans, drained and rinsed
1 14.5-ounce can Del Monte diced tomatoes with zesty mild green chilies
frozen corn—enough to fill the empty tomato can

Betsy wrote: "I just heated the ingredients together and served it with corn chips. The next day I added leftover polenta and oatmeal and made the recipe stretch."

Caribbean Black Beans with Mango Salsa over Brown Rice

MAKES 4 SERVINGS

The black beans are quick to prepare. The salsa (see below) takes some chopping, but the results are so fresh and delicious that it is worth every bit of effort.

1 large onion, chopped (1½ cups)
3 garlic cloves, minced or pressed
1–2 tablespoons peeled, grated, or chopped fresh ginger
1 teaspoon chopped fresh thyme, or ½ teaspoon dried
½ teaspoon ground allspice
3 15-ounce cans black beans, drained and rinsed
1 cup orange juice
pepper, to taste
mango salsa (recipe follows)

1. In a nonstick saucepan, stir-fry onions and garlic in a small amount of broth, water, wine, or other liquid for 5 minutes, until onions begin to soften.
2. Add ginger, thyme, and allspice and stir-fry 5 minutes more, until onions are very soft.
3. Stir in beans and orange juice and cook over low heat for about 15 minutes, stirring occasionally, until mixture thickens slightly. Mash a few beans with back of spoon for thicker consistency. Add pepper and serve over brown rice topped with mango salsa and crisped corn tortillas.

Mango Salsa

2 medium-size ripe mangos, peeled and chopped
1 small cucumber, peeled, seeded, and diced
1 ripe tomato, chopped (1 cup)
juice and zest of 1 lime
½–1 small fresh chili (jalapeño or other chili of your choice), minced, or hot pepper sauce, to taste
1 tablespoon (or more) chopped cilantro

Mix all ingredients and allow to stand for 10 minutes to allow flavors to blend.

Black Bean Cakes Supreme!

MAKES 8 SERVINGS

Our son-in-law, Brian Hart, made this delicious dish and we feasted on it—even our two- and four-year-old grandchildren, who loved helping to make the cakes.

BEAN CAKES:
6 15-ounce cans black beans, drained and rinsed
1 red bell pepper, seeded and chopped (1 cup)
3 green onions, chopped
2 carrots, grated
1 teaspoon garlic powder
1 teaspoon onion powder
1 teaspoon chili powder
2 teaspoons ground cumin
½ cup salsa

TOPPING:

1 16-ounce package frozen corn or kernels cut from 6 cobs
3 Vidalia onions, thinly sliced and slices cut in half
1 16-ounce jar salsa
1 bag spinach
½ cup chopped cilantro

1. Preheat oven to 350 degrees. Put beans in a large bowl. Add remaining bean cake ingredients, stirring to combine. Mash mixture well, using a potato masher or your hands.
2. Dump on a board or countertop and flatten into a circle about ½ inch thick. With a glass or biscuit cutter, form round cakes and put on a baking sheet.
3. Cover with aluminum foil and bake for 20 minutes. Remove foil and bake another 10 minutes, until tops are browned.
4. Roast corn on a baking sheet until browned. Put in a bowl.
5. Roast onions until browned. Put in a bowl.
6. Put bowls of corn, onions, bean cakes, salsa, spinach, and cilantro on the table. Start with spinach, then add a bean cake or two, roasted corn, roasted onions, and top with salsa and cilantro. If you do not have heart disease, you might want to add some avocado.

Fabulous Burritos

MAKES 4 SERVINGS

*Our sons Rip and Zeb surprised us one evening with this dish, which has become a family favorite. With a big salad, it makes a very satisfying meal. (**Note:** Ezekiel 4:9 sprouted grain tortillas, made by Food for Life, are especially good, and get crispy when heated. See Appendices I and II for product information.)*

1 large onion, chopped (1 cup)
2 garlic cloves, chopped

vegetable broth or water

2 15-ounce cans pinto beans, drained and rinsed

1–2 16-ounce jars mild salsa or no-oil pasta sauce or a combination of the two

4 no-oil whole-wheat thin flat bread or nonfat tortillas (the Ezekiel 4:9 tortillas are wonderful)

2–3 tomatoes or 6–8 plum tomatoes, thinly sliced

chopped cilantro or parsley

1. Preheat oven to 350 degrees.
2. In a nonstick saucepan, stir-fry onion and garlic in enough vegetable broth or water to cover until softened.
3. Add pinto beans and pasta sauce and mash (a potato masher works well), then cook for a few minutes. (If you want to expand this filling mixture, you could add leftover rice, corn, or other vegetables.)
4. Put enough pasta sauce in a baking pan just to cover the bottom. Spread each tortilla or piece of flat bread with bean mixture, roll up like a sausage, and place in the pan, nestling the burritos together. Cover rolled burritos with salsa, pasta sauce, or a combination of the two.
5. Place sliced tomatoes on top of the burritos.
6. Bake for 30 minutes, until bubbly, or more, if you like your burritos crispy. Sprinkle with chopped cilantro or parsley.

Jane's Burritos

MAKES 4–6 SERVINGS

Our daughter, Jane, serves this recipe often. She makes extras to freeze for later meals. We love her burrito meal! If freezing, bake first. Warm frozen burritos in 350-degree oven 10 minutes or until warmed through.

1 large onion, chopped (1 cup)

vegetable broth or water

2 small or 1 medium zucchini, chopped
2 small yellow squash, chopped
1 large red bell pepper, seeded and chopped (1 cup)
½ cup broccoli, chopped in tiny pieces
2 stalks bok choy, chopped
2 15-ounce cans vegetarian no-fat refried beans
1 15-ounce can pinto beans, drained and rinsed
2 cups brown rice, cooked
1 bunch cilantro, chopped
6 nonfat tortillas (Ezekiel 4:9 are good)
salsa

1. Preheat oven to 350 degrees.
2. Stir-fry onion in broth or water in a nonstick saucepan until limp. Add zucchini, squash, red pepper, broccoli, and bok choy and stir-fry 3–4 minutes, until just tender.
3. Stir in refried and pinto beans and cook 1 minute more.
4. Add as much rice as you like and stir in half of cilantro.
5. Put a few spoonfuls of mixture in each burrito. Fold one flap over mixture, then the other, and tilt each burrito a little on its side so that it leans into the next burrito to help keep it shut.
6. Bake for 12 minutes, or until tortillas are crispy. Serve with lots of salsa and remaining cilantro sprinkled on top.

Note: Use any vegetables you have in your refrigerator. Everything is good. The hardest part is finding a tortilla that is whole-grain and contains no fat. If you find some, load up your freezer, send away for a case, or ask your local health food store to carry your brand.

Very Quick Black Bean Chili

MAKES 4 SERVINGS

This is not only quick to make but also easy to eat. For an especially tasty meal, serve on a bed of steamed spinach topped with chopped green onions and crisped corn tortillas. If you're in a hurry, leave out the onions, use the garlic granules, wilt the spinach in the microwave—and presto!

1 large onion, chopped (1 cup)
2–3 garlic cloves, chopped, or 1 teaspoon garlic granules
2 15-ounce cans black beans, drained and rinsed
1 16-ounce jar salsa
1 bunch green onions, white and green parts, chopped
1 16-ounce package frozen corn (about 2 cups)
1/2–1 cup chopped cilantro

1. Stir-fry onion in a large nonstick saucepan over medium heat until soft and beginning to brown. Add garlic and continue cooking 1 minute longer.
2. Add beans, salsa, and green onions. Cover and cook over medium heat about 10 minutes, stirring occasionally.
3. Add corn and cook, stirring, until heated.
4. Add cilantro just before serving so that it stays green.

Easy Rice Chili

MAKES 6 SERVINGS

Lori Perry, the wife of a patient, sent this recipe—one of her favorites.

1 large yellow onion, chopped (1 cup)
2 ribs celery, chopped (1/2 cup)

1 jalapeño pepper, seeded and chopped
1 tablespoon minced garlic
1 14.5-ounce can low-sodium diced tomatoes
1 15-ounce can black beans, drained and rinsed
1 15-ounce can kidney beans, drained and rinsed
1 25.5-ounce jar oil-free spaghetti sauce
1 cup water
3/4 cup brown rice, uncooked
1 tablespoon chili powder
cilantro or parsley

1. In a nonstick pan, stir-fry onions, celery, jalapeño, and garlic in a small amount of water until cooked.
2. Add remaining ingredients except cilantro. Bring to a boil, then reduce heat and simmer, covered, approximately 1 hour, stirring frequently.
3. Add cilantro or parsley just before serving. Fill your bowl with greens and then add the chili or serve with a big green salad on the side.

Tortilla Pie

MAKES 4–6 SERVINGS

5–6 medium no-oil corn tortillas
2–3 15-ounce cans black beans, drained and rinsed
2 16-ounce jars salsa (mild or hotter, according to taste)
1 16-ounce package frozen corn
1 large onion, finely chopped (1 cup), and stir-fried until limp
1 large red or green bell pepper, seeded and chopped (1 cup)
1 large tomato, chopped (1 cup)

1. Preheat oven to 350 degrees.
2. Line bottom of a large baking dish with half of tortillas. You will need to cut or tear some in order to fit the pan.
3. Spread beans over tortillas, then add half the salsa, the corn, the stir-fried onions, peppers, tomato, and another layer of tortillas. Top with the rest of the salsa. Use extra salsa if necessary.
4. Bake for 60 minutes, uncovered. The longer it cooks, the better it tastes!

Broccoli-Mushroom Pie

MAKES 3–5 SERVINGS

1 teaspoon granulated garlic
1 teaspoon Mrs. Dash lemon pepper seasoning blend
2 cups brown rice, cooked
1 medium-large tomato, thinly sliced
1 bunch green onions, chopped
1 10-ounce box mushrooms, sliced
1 tablespoon miso
1 cup Lemon Sauce (see page 231)
3 cups broccoli, chopped and lightly steamed
1 bunch collard greens, stems removed, greens chopped in bite-size pieces, and steamed or boiled until soft
pepper, to taste

1. Preheat oven to 350 degrees.
2. Mix garlic and Mrs. Dash lemon pepper into cooked brown rice.
3. Cover bottom of a large pie plate with the cooked rice and pat into place.
4. Arrange tomato slices over rice and sprinkle with a handful of green onions.

5. In a nonstick saucepan, stir-fry mushrooms and remaining green onions in vegetable stock, wine, or water until just slightly cooked.
6. Mix miso in a small bowl with 2 tablespoons of stock or water, and stir into mushrooms.
7. Prepare Lemon Sauce.
8. Add broccoli and collards to the mushroom mixture, then mix in Lemon Sauce and pepper to taste.
9. Pour broccoli-mushroom mixture over tomatoes and bake for 20–30 minutes. (Optional: before baking, sprinkle lightly with nutritional yeast.)

Note: If you prefer, you can subsitute lightly steamed spinach or kale for collard greens.

Lemon Sauce

1 tablespoon whole-wheat flour
1 tablespoon cornstarch or arrowroot
1 tablespoon low-sodium tamari
1–2 tablespoons lemon juice plus zest of 1 lemon
pepper, to taste
1/2 cup vegetable broth
1/2 cup oat, almond, or nonfat soy milk

1. Combine first five ingredients in a saucepan.
2. Gradually add vegetable broth and milk, whisking until all lumps are gone.
3. Cook over medium heat, stirring constantly until sauce is smooth and thick.

Note: This sauce is also good with vegetables.

Ana's Amazing Vegetable Combination

MAKES 6 SERVINGS

Ana, who grew up in Lithuania on a plant-based diet, shared this unusual recipe which, as she says, "just works!" We agree.

1 large onion, chopped (1 cup)
vegetable broth, water, or wine
4 ribs celery, chopped (1 cup)
4 carrots, chopped
1 15-ounce can chickpeas, drained and rinsed
1 16-ounce package frozen peas, thawed under running water

1. In a nonstick saucepan, stir-fry onion in broth, water, or wine, until softened, then add celery and carrots.
2. Blend peas in a food processor until smooth.
3. Add chickpeas and blended pea mixture to onions. Stir, heat, and serve over brown rice or eat just plain.

Note: If almost any recipe needs thickening, blended frozen peas will do the trick. They are a magic ingredient!

Mushroom Ratatouille

MAKES 6–8 SERVINGS

This is absolutely delicious on top of brown rice, and best of all it's so easy!

2 large onions, chopped
3 garlic cloves, chopped, or more if you love garlic
16 ounces button mushrooms, large ones halved

7 ounces shiitake mushrooms, thickly sliced
1 eggplant, peeled and chopped into 1-inch pieces
3 tomatoes, chopped
1 teaspoon dried thyme
1 teaspoon dried basil
1 teaspoon pepper
1/2 cup vegetable broth or water
cilantro or parsley, chopped

1. Preheat oven to 375 degrees.
2. Place all ingredients except cilantro in a roasting pan or other pan with sides. Stir and cook uncovered for 50 minutes. If it cooks a little longer, dish is even better. If it gets a little dry, add a bit more broth or water. Before serving, stir in as much cilantro or parsley as you dare.

Note: If you do not have shiitake mushrooms, any variety works well in this recipe.

Barbecued Portobello Mushrooms

portobello mushrooms, 1–2 per person depending on size of mushrooms
barbecue sauce without oil or high-fructose corn syrup (or mix balsamic vinegar and no-oil tomato sauce for your own barbecue sauce)

1. Preheat oven to 350 degrees.
2. Cover mushrooms with barbecue sauce and place flat or slightly overlapping in a casserole dish. Add a small amount of water to pan.

3. Bake for at least 30 minutes—longer, if mushrooms are large. They must be soft.
4. Before serving, cover each mushroom with pan juices.

Note: These mushrooms are amazingly like meat. Serve with a grain, steamed vegetable, and a salad or put mushrooms on top of rice in a bowl, drizzle pan juices over rice, and surround with steamed or uncooked spinach. You may also put a barbecued portobello in a whole-grain bun (Alvarado Street Bakery and Food For Life both make good buns), or just use whole-grain bread. Add sliced tomato and lettuce and no-tahini hummus—or roasted red peppers, cilantro, and spinach. Fabulous!

Bright Summer Stir-fry

MAKES 4 SERVINGS

1 medium red onion, chopped (1/2 cup)
vegetable broth, water, wine, or orange juice
2 cups broccoli, cut in small pieces
2 ribs celery, sliced diagonally (1/2 cup)
1 red bell pepper, cut into thin strips
1 yellow summer squash, halved and cut into 1/2-inch slices
1 cup vegetable broth
4 ounces sugar snap peas
1 tablespoon peeled, minced fresh ginger
3 tablespoons low-sodium tamari or Bragg Liquid Aminos
1 tablespoon fresh lime juice
2 teaspoons cornstarch
2 tablespoons chopped cilantro (I always use *lots*!)

1. In a nonstick saucepan, stir-fry onion, adding liquid—broth, water, wine, or orange juice—as necessary, until onion begins to wilt.

2. Add broccoli, celery, peppers, and squash and cook about 5 minutes, until broccoli begins to soften, stirring constantly.
3. Stir in broth, sugar snap peas, and ginger and bring to a boil. Lower heat and simmer about 5 minutes, until vegetables are crisp-tender.
4. In a small bowl, stir together tamari, lime juice, and cornstarch.
5. Remove pan from heat and stir in tamari mixture. Return pan to medium heat and cook about 1 minute, until mixture boils and is slightly thickened, then stir in cilantro. Serve over brown rice.

Note: This is colorful and disappears quickly. You can substitute vegetables, if you wish—for example, green beans for sugar snap peas, cauliflower for broccoli.

Colorful Rice

MAKES 6–8 SERVINGS

1 very large or 2 medium portobello mushrooms, chopped
1 red onion, chopped
2–3 tablespoons Bragg Liquid Aminos or low-sodium tamari
1 16-ounce package frozen peas or mixed vegetables
4 cups cooked brown rice (about 2 cups uncooked)
chopped parsley
2 tablespoons chopped pimientos

1. Combine mushrooms and onion in a wok or nonstick pan and stir-fry about 5 minutes, until soft. Add 1–2 tablespoons Bragg Liquid Aminos or tamari, plus water if needed.
2. Add frozen vegetables and stir-fry until heated through.
3. Add rice and cook a few more minutes. Add parsley and another tablespoon of tamari or Bragg Liquid Aminos (according to taste) and top with pimientos.

Sweet Rice with Peas and Onions

MAKES 4 SERVINGS

1 red onion, chopped (1½ cups)
1 cup short-grain brown rice, uncooked
4 garlic cloves, crushed, or 2 teaspoons roasted garlic from a jar
1 16-ounce package frozen peas

1. Cook onion in a heavy, nonstick pan over high heat until softened, then reduce heat and simmer about 40 minutes. Add water and stir if necessary.
2. Cook brown rice in 2 cups of water in rice cooker or on the stovetop. It takes about 40 minutes either way.
3. Add garlic to onion just before rice is ready and stir-fry a few minutes.
4. Add rice to onion and garlic and stir.
5. Just before serving, add frozen peas and cook long enough to warm peas.

Note: The peas will keep their bright green color if you don't cook them too long. Even if you do, however, the dish is still deliciously sweet. Add cilantro before serving, if desired. This is good with a salad, baked portobello mushrooms, asparagus, and bread.

Rice with Salsa, Beans, and Cilantro

MAKES 2–3 SERVINGS

Guests we expected did not arrive, so we had leftover dip for hors d'oeuvres as well as leftover rice. Thus, this quick and surprisingly delicious combination.

1 16-ounce jar salsa
1 15-ounce can black beans, drained and rinsed
juice of 1/2 juicy lime or lemon
cilantro, lots

Mix all ingredients and serve over reheated rice.

Marvelous Wild Rice and Mushroom Pilaf

MAKES 6–8 SERVINGS

This is elegant enough for any special occasion and everyone *loves it! It is easy to make ahead.*

vegetable broth, water, or wine, or any other liquid for stir-frying
1 large onion or 2 medium onions, chopped (about 2 cups)
3 ribs celery, chopped (3/4 cup)
2 garlic cloves, minced
1 teaspoon dried thyme
3/4 cup wild rice
3/4 cup brown rice (we like the short-grain, but long is fine, too)
3 cups vegetable broth

2 10-ounce boxes fresh mushrooms, quartered
½ cup (or more) chopped parsley or cilantro
1–2 tablespoons balsamic vinegar
freshly ground black pepper, to taste

1. Heat a few tablespoons of vegetable broth, water, or wine, in a heavy casserole dish. Add onions and celery and cook 4–6 minutes, until soft, stirring often.
2. Add garlic and thyme and cook, stirring, for 30 seconds.
3. Add wild rice, brown rice, and vegetable broth and bring to a boil. Cover and simmer 50–55 minutes, until most of the liquid has been absorbed. There will be some liquid left in the pan.
4. Heat broth, water, or wine in a large nonstick pan over medium-high heat. Add mushrooms and cook 4–6 minutes, until browned and tender, stirring occasionally.
5. Add mushrooms to rice. Stir in parsley or cilantro, vinegar, and pepper. Fluff with a fork and feast!

Pineapple Stir-fry

MAKES 4–6 SERVINGS

1 large onion, chopped (1 cup)
3 garlic cloves, chopped
2 teaspoons peeled, chopped fresh ginger
1 10-ounce box mushrooms, sliced
2 red bell peppers, seeded and cut in 1-inch chunks
2 zucchini, sliced
3–4 leaves bok choy
1 fresh pineapple, diced
1 jalapeño pepper, seeded and chopped
2 tablespoons brown rice vinegar
pepper, to taste

1. In a nonstick saucepan, stir-fry onion, garlic, and ginger in pineapple juice, water, or vinegar until onion begins to soften.
2. Add mushrooms and cook a few minutes until the mushrooms begin to soften.
3. Add red peppers, zucchini, and bok choy and cook until warmed through and beginning to soften.
4. Mix pineapple, jalapeño, pepper, and vinegar in a small bowl and add to vegetables in saucepan. Cook until mixture is warmed through. Serve on top of brown rice or any favorite whole grain on a bed of greens.

Note: Almost any vegetables may be substituted. Use what you have!

Bok Choy, Mushroom, and Ginger Stir-fry

MAKES 4–6 SERVINGS

2 large onions, chopped (2 cups)
3 garlic cloves, minced
1½ tablespoons peeled, chopped fresh ginger
2 10-ounce boxes fresh mushrooms, sliced (about 4 cups)
8 stalks bok choy, white and green parts, chopped diagonally
6 green onions, chopped diagonally
1 large red bell pepper, seeded and chopped
½ cup water
3 tablespoons cornstarch
1–2 tablespoons low-sodium tamari or Bragg Liquid Aminos
black pepper, to taste
cilantro, lots, chopped
soba noodles or rice

1. In a nonstick pan, over medium-high heat, stir-fry onions, garlic, and ginger in vegetable broth, wine, or water for about 5 minutes, until onion begins to soften. Add mushrooms and cook 5 minutes.
2. Stir in bok choy and green onions. Cook for 2–3 minutes. Add red pepper.
3. Mix water, cornstarch, low-sodium tamari, or Bragg Liquid Aminos in a small bowl.
4. Lower heat to medium-low, stir in cornstarch mixture, cover, and cook a few minutes more, until liquid has thickened and glazed vegetables.
5. Add pepper and cilantro to taste and eat over soba noodles or rice—or just plain.

Swiss Chard with Garlic, Lemon, and Brown Rice

MAKES 2 SERVINGS

A neighbor gave me this recipe and said that she and her husband eat it at least once a week. Now we do, too!

vegetable broth, wine, or water
4 garlic cloves, chopped
1–2 bunches Swiss chard, chopped into 1- to 2-inch pieces (including stems) and washed
juice and zest of 1 lemon
2–3 cups cooked brown rice

1. Heat a little vegetable broth, wine, or water in a nonstick pan and add garlic. Stir for a minute, then add Swiss chard and more liquid, if necessary. Cook until the chard has wilted and reduced in size, stirring constantly.

2. Add lemon juice and zest, cook a minute more, then stir in cooked brown rice. Heat through and serve with a salad and bread.

Note: This is easy to make, and especially pretty if you use red Swiss chard, which turns the rice pink.

Swiss Chard and Chickpeas

MAKES 6 SERVINGS

Although it takes a bit of chopping, this dish is quicker than it seems—and is a meal in itself. The more Swiss chard you use, the better; go for more rather than less.

1 large red onion, chopped (1–1½ cups)
a pinch or two saffron threads
1 tablespoon chopped garlic
1 cup chopped cilantro
½ cup chopped parsley
½ teaspoon ground cumin
1 6-ounce can tomato paste
2 large bunches Swiss chard, leaves chopped and stems diced
2 15-ounce cans chickpeas, drained and rinsed
1 cup vegetable broth or water
black pepper, to taste

1. In a nonstick pan, over medium heat, stir-fry onions and saffron in broth, water, or wine about 10 minutes, until onions have softened.
2. Mix garlic, cilantro, parsley, and cumin in a bowl and add to onions along with tomato paste. Stir and cook over low heat for a few minutes.
3. Cook Swiss chard leaves first, in a few cups of water about 5 minutes, until wilted. Set leaves aside, reserving cooking water. Cook diced chard stems in same water about 10 minutes, until tender.

4. Add chickpeas, broth or water, and chard leaves to onion mixture. Simmer 10 minutes, then add stems and pepper to taste. Grated lemon zest and a squeeze of lemon on top add zip.

Veggie-Stuffed Peppers

MAKES 4–8 SERVINGS

4 bell peppers, any color
2 medium onions, chopped (1–1½ cups)
3 large garlic cloves, chopped
1 tablespoon peeled, chopped fresh ginger
broth, water, or wine (optional)
2 cups corn (about 3 ears)
2 cups cooked brown rice
2 medium tomatoes, chopped (2 cups)
1 tablespoon lemon juice and zest
1 tablespoon balsamic vinegar
pepper, to taste

1. Preheat oven to 400 degrees. Cut peppers in half lengthwise and remove seeds. Set peppers aside.
2. Stir-fry onions in a nonstick pan over medium heat until just beginning to brown.
3. Add garlic and ginger and continue stir-frying 2–3 minutes. Add broth, water, or wine if necessary.
4. Add corn and cook 2 minutes more.
5. Add rice, tomatoes, lemon juice, zest, vinegar, pepper and stir.
6. Fill pepper halves with vegetable mixture, pressing into corners of peppers and piling high.
7. Cover with aluminum foil and bake 25 minutes.

Note: You can also use this mixture to fill squash shells or hollowed-out cabbage—anything with a hole. Or you can eat it all by itself.

For a cheese-like effect, spread no-tahini hummus on top of the peppers and broil until browned.

Confetti Twice-Baked Potatoes

MAKES 6 SERVINGS

These are beautiful, and taste just as good as they look.

12 medium Yukon gold potatoes
2 cups or more oat or nonfat soy milk
1 16-ounce bag frozen corn
2 cups green chopped onions
2 large red bell peppers, seeded and chopped (2 cups)
1 teaspoon garlic granules or chopped fresh garlic
pepper, to taste

1. Preheat oven to 450 degrees.
2. Scrub potatoes, pierce with a knife, and bake for 1 hour.
3. Remove potatoes from the oven, carefully cut in half, scoop out insides into a large mixing bowl, and arrange skins in a baking dish.
4. Whip hot potatoes, adding milk slowly until quite soft.
5. Add corn, green onions, red peppers, garlic, and pepper. Mix well.
6. Lower oven temperature to 350 degrees and bake for 30 minutes.

Note: Our grandchildren liked these with just the oat milk and even ate the skins. Leftovers, if there are any, heat well in the microwave or can be frozen. For variety, bake a butternut squash along with potatoes and mix the squash insides with potatoes and green onions. The squash gives the potatoes a slightly sweet taste and a lovely color. For other variations, add almost any vegetable: grated carrot, chopped broccoli, chopped red peppers, peas, lima beans, cilantro, parsley—or all of the above.

Mashed Potatoes

MAKES 4 SERVINGS

4 large russet/Idaho potatoes, or 6–8 Yukon gold potatoes (although Yukon gold are not as fluffy as russet/Idaho, they have more flavor, even a buttery taste)
½ cup oat, nonfat soy milk, or potato water
1 teaspoon granulated onion
½–1 teaspoon granulated garlic
⅛ teaspoon black pepper

1. Cut potatoes into 6–8 pieces. Peeling is optional. I rarely peel potatoes for any reason.
2. Place potatoes in a pot with water to cover. Place pot over medium-high heat and bring to a rolling boil. (Alternatively, bake, instead of boiling, for a more intense flavor.)
3. Continue boiling potatoes 20–25 minutes, until they are soft, but not mushy.
4. Drain potatoes, saving water if using. Return to pot and shake, over medium heat, 2–3 minutes, to dry. Transfer to bowl of an electric mixer or use a hand mixer. Beat potatoes on high speed for 1 minute. (The hotter the potatoes, the less likely you are to end up with lumps.)
5. Turn mixer to low speed and slowly add milk or water. Scrape sides of bowl.
6. Add seasonings and beat again on high for 1 minute. Serve plain or with Mushroom Gravy (see Chapter 18). Leftover mashed potatoes make good potato pancakes "fried" in a nonstick pan. (**Note:** To prevent water-logging, put ¼ lemon in the cooking water and boil the potatoes with skins on.)

Potato "Fries"

These are so good, plain or with ketchup, you will find yourself eating more than you can believe. Don't make too many!

potatoes, red or white, sliced thin, 1 large or 2–3 medium per person
low-sodium tamari or Bragg Liquid Aminos

1. Preheat oven to 350 degrees.
2. Arrange potatoes on a baking sheet, spray with tamari or Bragg Liquid Aminos, and bake for 30 minutes—longer, if you like them crispy.

Deviled Baby Potatoes

MAKES 6 SERVINGS

These are excellent cold, as hors d'oeuvres, or hot or cold as the centerpiece of a meal. Our grandchildren love eating the scooped-out potato balls.

1. Steam 12 small red potatoes for about 20 minutes, then plunge them into cold water in a big bowl. Chill.
2. Slice each potato in half. Using the small end of a melon baller or a small spoon, scoop out a hole in the center.
3. Fill each hole with Hummus and Green Onion Sauce (see page 246), Sweet Corn Sauce or Walnut Sauce (see Chapter 18), mustard, or some other sauce of your choice.
4. Top with a few parsley or cilantro leaves and serve.

Hummus and Green Onion Sauce

10 tablespoons ($^1/_2$ cup plus 2 tablespoons) no-tahini hummus
$^1/_2$ cup chopped green onions, white and green parts
2 teaspoons Dijon mustard

Mix all ingredients until combined.

Layered Mashed White and Sweet Potatoes with Greens

MAKES 10 SERVINGS

This delicious recipe has been adapted from CalciYum! *by David and Rochelle Bronfman. It is attractive and flavorful, well worth the fuss of chopping and steaming!*

6 medium white potatoes, peeled and cut into 1-inch chunks (if you don't mind skins, don't peel)
$^3/_4$–1 cup oat, or nonfat soy milk
2 medium sweet potatoes, peeled and chunked
1 large onion, chopped (1 cup)
4 cups packed collard greens, finely chopped and steamed
3 cups chopped Napa cabbage, steamed (about $^1/_2$ cabbage)
$^1/_4$ cup finely chopped fennel (not necessary to steam)
cilantro, chopped

1. Cook white potatoes in a large pot of boiling water until soft. Drain and transfer to a large bowl. Mash, adding milk, until no longer stiff.
2. Steam or boil sweet potatoes until soft. Drain, and transfer to another large bowl.

3. Stir-fry onions in a nonstick pan over medium-high heat until brown, adding water or broth as necessary. Add onions to mashed white potatoes along with collard greens. Mix well.
4. Add cabbage and fennel to sweet potatoes. Mix well.
5. Put a single layer of white potatoes in a 9 × 11-inch baking dish. Follow with a layer of sweet potatoes. Finish with a layer of white potatoes.
6. Preheat oven to 350 degrees.
7. Bake for 30 minutes. Sprinkle with chopped cilantro and devour!

Whole-Wheat Pasta with Roasted Vidalia Onions and Diced Tomatoes

MAKES 6 SERVINGS

4 large Vidalia or sweet onions, thinly sliced
1 16-ounce package whole-wheat angel hair pasta or whole-grain pasta of your choice
4 14.5-ounce cans diced tomatoes (Contadina brand is a rich, thick sauce quite low in sodium.)
$^{1}/_{4}$ cup (or more) chopped basil, cilantro, or parsley

1. Turn oven on broil.
2. Spread onions on a baking sheet and put in the oven. Broil, checking every few minutes, until the onions are brown and very limp. Turn and brown more. If they get a little burned, they will still taste delicious.
3. While the onions are broiling, cook pasta according to package directions.
4. Put diced tomatoes in a casserole dish and heat on stove top until just beginning to bubble.
5. Add cooked pasta, stir, and heat.

6. Cover the pasta with fresh basil and top with the roasted onions. Do not mix the onions into the pasta. Serve with whole-grain bread and a salad full of vegetables. You will be in heaven! You can cut this recipe in half for two, but be careful not to use too much pasta. It needs lots of sauce and plenty of onions.

Note: It is often hard to find no-oil pasta sauce. This is easy, quick, and surprisingly delicious simply with diced tomatoes. For variety, roast garlic with the onions or add steamed broccoli florets at the end.

Whole-Grain Pasta with Greens, Beans, and Tomato Sauce

MAKES 4–6 SERVINGS

This is a meal in one dish. Cooking kale, collards, or Swiss chard along with pasta is an easy way to prepare those greens and there is no limit to the amount of greens you can use. In fact, more greens than pasta would be perfect! If you have a no-oil pasta sauce, you can use that instead of diced tomatoes and tomato sauce. As always, fresh basil is by far the best.

1 large onion, chopped (1 cup)
3–4 garlic cloves, chopped
1 15-ounce can no-salt-added tomatoes, diced
1 15-ounce can no-oil tomato sauce
1 15- to 19-ounce can cannellini beans, drained and rinsed
1 teaspoon dried oregano
lots of fresh basil, or 1 teaspoon dried basil
black pepper
12 ounces whole-wheat, spelt, or quinoa pasta
1 bunch kale, collards, or Swiss chard, stems removed and chopped into bite-size pieces
cilantro

1. Bring a large pot of water to a boil.
2. Stir-fry onion in a nonstick pan over medium heat until wilted and beginning to brown, adding water as necessary. Add garlic and stir-fry a few minutes more.
3. Add diced tomatoes, tomato sauce, beans, oregano, and basil and simmer uncovered 10–15 minutes. Add pepper to taste.
4. Add pasta to the boiling water and cook a few minutes, then add greens and stir into the pasta. Cook 5 minutes longer, or until pasta is cooked. Drain well. Transfer to a casserole dish or bowl and stir in the sauce. Sprinkle cilantro on top and dig in!

Sloppy Lentil Joes

MAKES 8–10 SERVINGS

This is Mary McDougall's recipe, slightly adapted. We found it very flavorful, and like it best by itself, with steamed spinach or kale and a big salad, although it is also good served on whole-grain buns or over rice.

3¹/₃ cups water
1 large onion, chopped (1 cup)
1 bell pepper—any color—seeded and chopped (1 cup)
1 tablespoon chili powder
1¹/₂ cups dried lentils, red or brown
1 15-ounce can crushed or diced tomatoes
1 tablespoon low-sodium tamari or Bragg Liquid Aminos
2 tablespoons mustard, Dijon or your choice
1 tablespoon brown sugar (optional)
1 tablespoon rice vinegar
1 teaspoon vegetarian Worcestershire sauce
1 bunch cilantro, chopped
freshly ground black pepper, to taste

1. Place $^1/_3$ cup water in a large pot. Add onions and bell pepper and cook about 5 minutes, until onions soften slightly, stirring occasionally.
2. Add chili powder and mix well.
3. Add remaining water, the lentils, tomatoes, and the rest of the ingredients. Mix well, bring to a boil, lower heat, cover, and cook over low heat for 55 minutes, stirring occasionally.

Sweet-and-Sour Seitan with Vegetables

MAKES 6 SERVINGS

Lori Perry, the wife of a patient, suggested this recipe for her vegetarian club to serve one night when Essy spoke to them. It was delicious, served over brown rice with broccoli and cauliflower on the side. Seitan is made from wheat gluten and looks like meat!

2 teaspoons plus 2 tablespoons low-sodium tamari or Bragg Liquid Aminos
8 ounces seitan, cut into cubes
2 cups broccoli florets, lightly steamed
1 large sweet onion, sliced and slices halved
1 cup grated carrots (packaged matchstick carrots are easy)
1 large red bell pepper, seeded and cut into strips
3–4 garlic cloves, crushed
2 teaspoons peeled, grated fresh ginger
1 16-ounce can crushed pineapple packed in juice
$^1/_4$ cup apple cider vinegar
1 tablespoon sweetener of your choice (optional)
1 tablespoon cornstarch
2 green onions, thinly sliced
cooked brown rice

1. Heat 2 teaspoons tamari or Bragg Liquid Aminos in a large nonstick pan. When hot, add seitan and cook until browned all over, stirring constantly. Add more tamari or water if necessary. Remove to a separate bowl.
2. Stir-fry broccoli florets in same pan, until just tender, adding water as necessary. Remove to a separate bowl.
3. Stir-fry onions until browned, adding broth or water, if necessary.
4. Add carrots, peppers, garlic, and ginger and stir-fry until peppers are tender. Add more water if necessary.
5. Drain pineapple, reserving the juice. Combine juice, vinegar, sweetener (optional), cornstarch, and 2 tablespoons tamari or Bragg Liquid Aminos in a small bowl or measuring cup. Whisk until well combined.
6. Add seitan and broccoli to other vegetables. Pour whisked ingredients over seitan and vegetables, then add pineapple chunks. Heat, stirring constantly, until sauce is just thickened, about 2 minutes.
7. Garnish with sliced green onions and serve over brown rice.

Note: This is a little fussy, but worth the effort. Do not overcook. It is possible to assemble all ingredients ahead through Step 5, then combine everything else just before serving. Possible additions or substitutes: mushrooms, sliced zucchini, spinach.

Seitan Bourguignon

MAKES 6–8 SERVINGS

3 medium onions, chopped (1½ cups)
12 ounces mushrooms, sliced
2 cups cubed seitan
1 cup red wine
1½ cups vegetable broth
⅓ cup low-sodium tamari or Bragg Liquid Aminos

1/4 teaspoon dried marjoram
1/4 teaspoon dried thyme
1/8 teaspoon ground black pepper
2 1/2 tablespoons cornstarch mixed with 1/4 cup water
cilantro or parsley

1. Stir-fry onions and mushrooms in 1/2 cup water in a nonstick pan for about 15 minutes, or until onions are tender.
2. Add remaining ingredients except for cornstarch mixture and simmer 5 minutes.
3. Add cornstarch mixture and cook, stirring until thickened.

Note: If you can find fat-free veggie burgers, crumble them and use them instead of or along with the seitan. This is *delicious* on rice, over potatoes, on whole-wheat toast, over millet—or even alone! Double or triple mushrooms, if desired. More seitan is good, too.

Antonia Demas's Couscous and African Stew

MAKES 8 SERVINGS

Antonia Demas is a well-known chef who has done pioneering work teaching children and adults how to eat a plant-based diet. This dish is quick, especially if you cook the sweet potato ahead of time. It freezes well and you can add more corn and tomatoes to expand leftovers. But there won't be many with this delicious dish.

2 cups whole-wheat couscous
1 large onion, chopped (1 cup)
1 large green bell pepper, seeded and chopped (1 cup)
2 cups chopped carrots
2 tablespoons ground cumin
2 tablespoons paprika

1 tablespoon ground cinnamon
2 medium tomatoes, diced (2 cups)
2 cups green beans (fresh or frozen, any style)
2 cups baked sweet potatoes (1 large or 2 small)
1 15-ounce can chickpeas, drained and rinsed
2 cups fresh or frozen green peas
2 cups (or less) raisins
Tabasco, to taste

1. Bring 2 cups of water to a boil and add couscous. Stir and remove from heat. Let stand, covered, for at least 5 minutes.
2. Stir-fry onion in a nonstick pan a few minutes, then add green pepper and water as necessary.
3. Add carrots, cumin, paprika, and cinnamon. Stir-fry a few minutes, then add tomatoes, beans, sweet potatoes, and chickpeas; cook over medium heat about 15 minutes.
4. Add peas and raisins and heat briefly, then add Tabasco, if desired. Serve over couscous.

Lentil Loaf

MAKES 6 SERVINGS

Any lentils will work in this healthy loaf, but my favorite is red lentils, which cook and mash quickly and make a lighter-colored loaf. If brown lentils don't mash easily, add a little water and cook a few minutes longer. Leftovers make a great sandwich—or you can "fry" slices in a nonstick pan.

1½ cups lentils, rinsed
2½ cups water
2 medium onions, chopped (1½ cups)
6 mushrooms, chopped
2 cups packed fresh spinach, chopped
1 15-ounce can diced tomatoes

- 2 cups brown rice, cooked
- 1 teaspoon garlic powder
- 1 teaspoon dried sage
- 1 teaspoon Mrs. Dash's garlic and herb seasoning blend
- 1/2 teaspoon dried marjoram
- 1/4–1/2 cup ketchup or barbecue sauce

1. Preheat oven to 350 degrees.
2. Cook lentils in 2 1/2 cups water until tender, then partially mash lentils in the cooking water.
3. Stir-fry onions and mushrooms in broth or water in a nonstick pan. Add spinach and cook, covered, until spinach wilts.
4. Add onions and mushrooms, tomatoes, rice, garlic, sage, Mrs. Dash, and marjoram to lentils.
5. Press into a 9 × 5-inch loaf pan and spread ketchup or barbecue sauce on top.
6. Bake uncovered for 45–60 minutes. Serve with mashed potatoes, Mushroom Gravy (see Chapter 18), and salad.

Note: Look for barbecue sauce or ketchup without high-fructose corn syrup. Examples: Bone Suckin' Sauce Thicker Style and Muir Glen ketchup.

Mustard Seed Quinoa

MAKES 6–8 SERVINGS

- 1 tablespoon black mustard seeds
- 2 cups quinoa, rinsed
- 3 1/2 cups water
- 2 large (or more) onions, sliced and slices halved
- 1 tablespoon low-sodium tamari or Bragg Liquid Aminos
- 1/4–1 cup (or more) chopped cilantro or parsley
- pinch of cayenne

1. Place mustard seeds in a small, hot pan. Have a lid ready to cover seeds once they begin to pop. Turn off heat after seeds begin to pop and remove pan from heat.
2. Bring water to a boil in a medium pan. Add quinoa, cover, and cook over low heat for 15 minutes.
3. While quinoa cooks, turn oven to broil. Put halved onion slices on a baking sheet and broil, watching closely. Turn as onions begin to brown. They need to be brown and wilted—and they taste just as good if some get burned.
4. When quinoa is cooked, add mustard seeds, low-sodium tamari or Bragg Liquid Aminos, cilantro, and cayenne. Stir, put in an 8 × 12-inch pan, and top with the browned onions. *Don't stir the onions in.* The onions are what make this dish, so make certain they are spread out, and every bite will be topped with onions.

Curried Chickpeas with Chutney

MAKES 3–4 SERVINGS

This is very quick and looks pretty served on a bed of arugula or baby spinach.

1 15-ounce can chickpeas, drained and rinsed
3 medium ripe tomatoes, diced (or 2 14.5-ounce cans diced tomatoes)
2 teaspoons curry powder, or to taste
1 8- or 9-ounce jar sweet and spicy mango chutney, or 1 fresh mango, chopped
2 cups cooked short-grain brown rice, or 1¼ cups cooked bulgur
chopped cilantro—lots!

1. In a saucepan, combine chickpeas, tomatoes, and curry powder. Bring to a simmer over medium heat and cook 3–4 minutes. Cover until ready to use.
2. Stir chutney or chopped mango into cooked rice or bulgur.

3. Just before serving, add chopped cilantro to rice mixture. Mound rice or bulgur on each plate and top with the chickpea mixture.

Note: Trader Joe's makes a good version of Major Grey's Mango Chutney. If you want to avoid sugar, use chopped mango, raisins, and a little vinegar, a good no-sugar apple butter, or chopped mango all by itself.

Cauliflower and Potato Curry

MAKES 6 SERVINGS

I love this dish!

1½ cups onion (about 1 large onion), thinly sliced
3 teaspoons minced fresh ginger
2–3 tablespoons vegetable broth or wine
1 tablespoon curry powder
3 cloves garlic, minced (about 3 teaspoons)
4 cups cauliflower florets
1½ pounds red potatoes (about 4 medium), cubed
1 28-ounce can diced tomatoes
1 package frozen peas
½ cup chopped cilantro

1. Put onion, ginger and vegetable broth or wine in a casserole dish on medium high. Cover and cook about 4 minutes.
2. Reduce heat to medium. Add curry powder and garlic and cook about a minute, stirring constantly.
3. Add cauliflower and potatoes and cook, stirring often, 5 minutes or until they begin to soften.
4. Add tomatoes, reduce heat and cook covered 15 minutes or until vegetables are tender.
5. Stir in peas and cook covered until peas are warm, about 2 minutes.
6. Add cilantro, stir, and serve with a salad and bread.

Easy, Easy Curried Rice with Raisins

MAKES 3–4 SERVINGS

I love this dish. Best of all, it takes just a little chopping—and it cooks by itself.

1 cup brown rice, uncooked
1½ cups vegetable broth
½ cup orange juice
2 tablespoons orange zest
1½ teaspoons curry powder
1½ teaspoons ground cumin
1 large bell pepper, any color, seeded and chopped (1 cup)
1 medium onion, chopped (¾ cup)
¼ cup raisins
chopped parsley or cilantro
1 fresh mango or peach, chopped

1. Put rice, broth, orange juice, zest, curry powder, cumin, pepper, and onion in a rice cooker or covered pot and cook about 40 minutes, until rice is done.
2. Add raisins when rice is just cooked. Stir and let stand a few minutes so raisins plump up.
3. Add parsley. Serve topped with chopped mango or peach or eat as is with steamed broccoli or greens. You can't feast in an easier way!

Note: If fresh mangos or peaches are not available, substitute mango chutney.

Curried Chickpeas with Spinach in a Pressure Cooker

MAKES 4–6 SERVINGS

This takes almost no time and is so good that it makes buying a pressure cooker worthwhile. Serve over rice, with mango chutney or chopped fresh mangos on the side.

2 cups vegetable broth or water
1 cup oat, almond, or nonfat soy milk
2 tablespoons mild curry powder
1 pound (2½ cups) dried chickpeas, soaked overnight in water to cover
2 10-ounce packages frozen chopped spinach
2 large red onions, peeled and cut into eighths
1 15-ounce can diced tomatoes with chilies, including liquid, or 1 15-ounce can diced tomatoes
chopped cilantro—lots!

1. Blend broth, milk, and curry powder in a pressure cooker.
2. Drain chickpeas and add to the pot.
3. Set frozen blocks of spinach and onions on top of chickpeas.
4. Pour tomatoes over spinach and onions.
5. Following the safety instructions for your pressure cooker, cook the ingredients on high for 18 minutes.
6. Stir well. Curry will thicken as it stands, but if you wish to thicken immediately, mash some chickpeas against the side of cooker with a fork and stir them in.
7. Garnish individual portions with cilantro or just sprinkle the whole pot with lots.

Indian Dahl

MAKES 4 SERVINGS

I learned this from a superb cook in Bombay. I omit the salt. The three last ingredients are my additions. 1 tablespoon chopped fresh ginger in step 2 is another good addition.

2½ cups yellow lentils (red lentils or yellow peas also work)
5 cups water
4 garlic cloves, chopped
1 onion, chopped (1 cup)
1 tomato, chopped (½ cup)
4 skinny green chili peppers (1 jalapeño, 2 or 3 green mild chilies, or some combination, depending on taste), chopped and seeds removed
1 teaspoon salt (optional)
1 teaspoon ground turmeric
cilantro
shredded carrots
chopped red peppers
chopped zucchini

1. Combine lentils and water, bring to a boil, lower heat, and cook 10 minutes until lentils soften.
2. Add garlic, onion, tomato, chilies, and turmeric to the lentils, and simmer, uncovered, until mixture is smooth and onion is soft.
3. Add remaining ingredients at the last minute, and serve over brown rice on a big bed of steamed spinach and green salad.

Slow-Cooker Dahl

MAKES 6 SERVINGS

Our daughter, Jane, came home from dinner at a friend's and said she had had the best dahl, and it contained only a few ingredients. I called to check, and Peter, the cook, gave me the following easy recipe. The ginger makes it!

2 large yellow onions, chopped (2 cups)
9 garlic cloves, chopped
7 tablespoons peeled, chopped fresh ginger
7 cups broth or water
1 16-ounce package yellow peas

1. Stir-fry onions in a nonstick pan until translucent, using water or broth as necessary. Add garlic and ginger and stir-fry until onions begin to brown.
2. Put 7 cups of yellow peas and onion mixture in slow cooker and cook for 6–10 hours, until the mixture is smooth. Serve over brown rice with steamed spinach or kale around it.

Note: If you don't have a slow cooker, simmer on the stove top for as long as it takes for the mixture to become smooth.

Kitchari

MAKES 10 SERVINGS

We adapted this from a dish we tasted at the 2004 Boston Vegetarian Society. It was made by Hare Krishnas from Iskcon Temple, who generously handed out samples—and recipe cards. Kitchari is considered an Indian comfort food, and we understand why. Asafoetida, available in health food stores, is a delicious Indian and Iranian spice worth finding, but this recipe works without it, too.

1 cup yellow split peas
2 cups brown rice, uncooked
1 large sweet potato, cubed (2 cups)
1 small head cauliflower, chopped into bite-size pieces (2 cups)
1½ teaspoons ground turmeric
1 tablespoon cumin seeds
2 jalapeño peppers, seeded and finely chopped
1 teaspoon asafoetida
4 teaspoons peeled, grated fresh ginger
1 heaping tablespoon white miso (optional)
freshly ground black pepper, to taste
spinach
lots of cilantro, chopped

1. Cook peas in 12 cups of water about 10 minutes, until soft but not broken down.
2. Add rice, sweet potatoes, cauliflower, and turmeric and cook until softened.
3. Stir-fry cumin seeds in a small, hot frying pan until slightly darkened, shaking pan constantly and watching closely so cumin doesn't burn.
4. Add jalapeño peppers and ginger and stir-fry for a few seconds, adding water if necessary.
5. Add spice mixture and asafoetida to peas and cook over low heat for about 45 minutes. Add optional miso and pepper and stir.
6. To serve, put a handful of spinach in a bowl, add hot kitchari, and top with chopped cilantro and you have a meal. Kitchari is especially good if spinach wilts, so add it to pot just before serving, to individual bowl if kitchari is HOT, or zap spinach and kitchari in a microwave. Add more liquid if you don't want kitchari so thick, and Tabasco or other hot sauce to taste if you find it too bland. Sleep well!

Pasta Toppers

It is helpful to find a ready-made pasta sauce you like, but it is also fun to make your own, especially in the summer and fall, when tomatoes are plentiful and delicious. The following varieties are easy to prepare.

Easy Basil Pasta Sauce

MAKES ABOUT 4 CUPS

Start this first, and it will be ready by the time the rest of the dinner is headed for the table.

1 large onion, chopped (1 cup)
5–6 garlic cloves, chopped
1 28-ounce can crushed low-sodium tomatoes
1 6-ounce can no-salt-added tomato paste
½ cup wine (optional)
1 teaspoon dried oregano
lots of fresh basil (1–2 cups, chopped)
black pepper, to taste

1. Stir-fry onion in broth, water, or wine until beginning to brown. Add garlic and continue to cook a few minutes more.
2. Add crushed tomatoes, tomato paste, wine, oregano, basil, and pepper.
3. Simmer, uncovered, about 20 minutes, stirring often. Continue cooking for 10 minutes, until thickened, or until the pasta is ready and you are too impatient to wait.
4. Add 2 tablespoons of pasta water to sauce before spooning over pasta.

VARIATION:
Add sliced mushrooms in Step 2 or diced peppers in Step 3. Always add spinach, when possible, either in the sauce just before you serve it or on the side.

Roasted Plum Tomato Pasta Sauce

MAKES 2–4 SERVINGS

1. Preheat oven to 350 degrees.
2. Cut 20–30 plum tomatoes in half and place cut side up on a baking sheet.
3. Bake for 1–2 hours. They get sweeter the longer they bake. If they get black, they are still good—maybe even better!
4. Transfer shriveled tomatoes to a blender and process until smooth (although they taste so good, you may eat a lot of them before they make the blender!).

Roasted Tomatoes and Garlic Pasta Sauce

MAKES 2–4 SERVINGS

6–7 tomatoes, cut in half
2 heads of garlic, tops cut off
2–3 tablespoons red wine vinegar
pepper, to taste
lots of fresh basil

1. Preheat oven to 375 degrees.
2. Place tomatoes and garlic on a baking sheet, and bake for 30 minutes.
3. Carefully pour off tomato juices into a bowl and set aside. Return tomatoes to oven and bake another 30 minutes.

4. Remove from oven and let cool. Remove tomato skins and squeeze garlic out of cloves. Combine tomatoes and garlic in a blender, and process until smooth.
5. Stir in vinegar, pepper, and basil. If you want to thin the sauce, add reserved juices.

Susie and Judy's Sinfully Good Roasted Tomatoes

My sister, Susie, always has good cooking ideas. She and a friend presented us with a beautiful bowl of roasted tomatoes—and this recipe.

20 tomatoes, any type, cut in half, with a little juice squeezed out of the larger tomatoes and reserved
3–4 slices whole-grain bread, toasted and crumbled
4 garlic cloves, chopped
$^1/_4$–$^1/_3$ cup chopped chives, green onions, or shallots

1. Preheat oven to 300 degrees.
2. Roast tomatoes for 2 hours. Turn off oven and let sit for an hour. (If you are in a hurry, simply cook the tomatoes an additional 30 minutes.) Remove from oven.
3. Mix crumbled bread with garlic and chives. Add reserved tomato juice and mix again until moistened but not runny. Sprinkle bread mixture on tomato halves and bake for 45 minutes.
4. Place each roasted tomato on a piece of toast or a cracker and serve as an amazing hors d'oeuvre, or put on top of pasta, rice, or baked potatoes. For the best treat of all, just eat each little tomato one bite at a time. They are sweet and addicting.

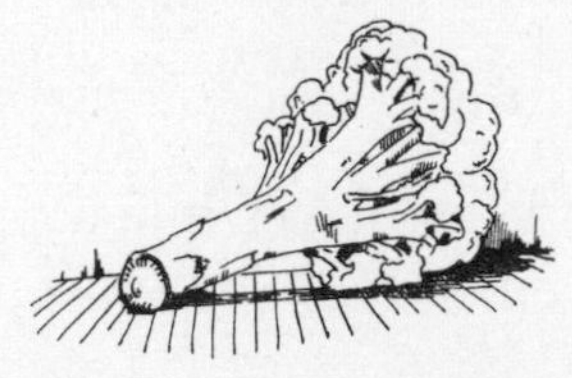

23

Wonderful, Easy Desserts

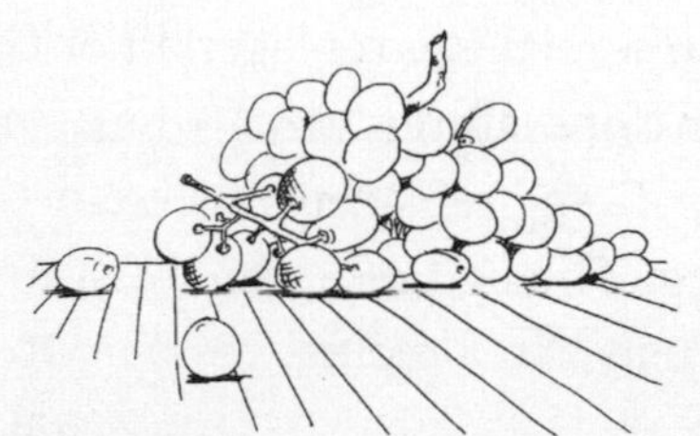

IT IS BEST NOT TO EAT DESSERT every night. Make it a rare treat, when there will be lots of people around—and no temptation to eat too much!

Freeze grapes, pineapple, or banana slices for times when you want to snack on a sweet, cold treat. A bowl of "iced" grapes on the table after dinner makes everyone feel satisfied. The best dessert of all is a matter of freezing fruits and, using a juicer or food processor, causing a magical transformation to "ice cream" (see Magic Banana "Ice Cream," page 267).

In baking, try using some of your own recipes with the following changes:

- Reduce the amount of sugar you use as much as possible. Consider using agar nectar instead of sugar.

- Use whole-grain flours instead of white flour. Try whole-wheat, barley, or spelt flour.

- Replace cow's milk with oat, almond, or nonfat soy milk.

- Instead of oil, use equal amounts of applesauce or prunes (baby-food prunes are easy).

- Instead of eggs, use 1 tablespoon flaxseed meal plus 3 tablespoons water for each egg called for in a recipe. (Buy flaxseed meal already ground and keep it refrigerated or in the freezer, or buy whole flaxseeds and grind them yourself.) Mix the flaxseed meal and the water until frothy and use as if it were an egg, or take the lazy way out: simply add the ground flax to the liquid ingredients in the recipe. (Be sure to increase the liquid ingredients by 3 tablespoons per tablespoon of flaxseed meal.) If you prefer to use a commercial egg replacer, Ener-G egg replacer, available at health food stores, works best in baked goods; 1½ teaspoons Ener-G egg replacer plus 2 tablespoons warm water equals 1 egg. The egg replacer must be beaten with a liquid before you use it in a recipe.

Baked goods cooked with these substitutes will not be as light and may be more moist than those you used to produce, but they will taste every bit as good. And there's a delicious bonus, as well: you know they will not harm you.

Note: Nonstick baking pans make life much easier when you're cooking without fat. But you can use old-fashioned pans, too; you may need to spray lightly with Pam, wipe with paper towels, and dust lightly with flour before adding batter.

Magic Banana "Ice Cream"

1 ripe banana per person (the riper the banana, the sweeter the "ice cream")

1. Peel and slice bananas, place on a baking sheet, and freeze.
2. Remove from freezer and thaw slightly—enough so that you can remove slices from baking sheet.
3. Place frozen bananas in a strong blender or juicer. We use a Champion juicer exclusively to make this dessert. If you are using a blender, thaw slices a little longer to avoid overtaxing the appliance.
4. Sprinkle with ground nutmeg or cinnamon, then add a little vanilla extract, a few Grape-Nuts, berries, maple syrup—or all of the above. You might even put some chocolate sauce on top (see following recipe). But this dessert is so good, it needs nothing! Frozen mangos are especially good in this recipe (and it is worth noting that Trader Joe's sells bags of frozen mangos—ready to use). You can also try frozen berries or a combination of frozen fruits. Experiment to see what you like.

Chocolate Sauce

MAKES ABOUT ½ CUP

3 tablespoons maple syrup, honey, agar nectar, or sugar
2 tablespoons unsweetened cocoa powder
½ cup water
1 teaspoon cornstarch or arrowroot
1 teaspoon vanilla extract

In a saucepan, combine sugar, cocoa, water, cornstarch, and vanilla. Mix well and cook over medium heat until thickened, stirring constantly. Use for dipping whole strawberries or drizzle over berries or any other fruit. It is positively delicious over broiled bananas.

Skewered Fruit with Lovely Lime Sauce

This is delicious and refreshing any time of year, and so *pretty. Find other combinations of fruit, if you like. Everything is good.*

fresh pineapple, cut in chunks
kiwi, thickly sliced
strawberries, hulled
cantaloupe, cut in chunks

SAUCE:
1 12.3-ounce box light firm tofu
3 tablespoons maple syrup (or other sweetener of choice)
3 tablespoons fresh lime juice, plus lime zest to taste

1. Arrange fruit on bamboo skewers and put in a shallow bowl, with one end sticking out.
2. Put tofu, maple syrup, lime juice, and zest in a blender. Blend well, scraping down sides of container. Blend again. Place in one large bowl or several small bowls, and dip fruit in sauce.

Sliced Strawberries and Balsamic Vinegar or Vanilla

This is especially good if the strawberries available are not at their stand-alone best.

Wash, hull, and slice strawberries. Sprinkle with a little balsamic vinegar or vanilla. Mix well. Serve alone or over banana "ice cream." Top with a sprinkling of sugar if not sweet enough. (It may seem surprising, but balsamic vinegar is wonderful with some fruits; try it sprinkled on quartered figs!)

Summer Fruit with Lime and Mint

MAKES 6–8 SERVINGS

1 melon (cantaloupe, honeydew, or Crenshaw—or a combination)
3/4 cup fresh raspberries
3/4 cup fresh blueberries
1 teaspoon lime zest
juice of 1 lime
6–8 mint leaves, shredded

1. Cut melon into 1/2-inch pieces (or use a melon baller) and place in a bowl.
2. Scatter raspberries and blueberries over melon.
3. Sprinkle zest over fruit and squeeze lime juice over top, then spread mint leaves over fruit.

Stunning Grilled Pineapple

Our niece stunned us all at a Fourth of July barbecue when she covered the grill with large slices of pineapple. The seared, juicy result was a remarkably delicious surprise for all of us!

Peel, core, and slice 1 pineapple. Grill in the oven or outside until each slice has grill marks. Flip, and grill the other side. You will never want to eat pineapple another way.

Grapefruit and Orange Slices with Mint and Lime

MAKES 6 SERVINGS

4 grapefruit, preferably 2 white and 2 pink
4 oranges
6 mint leaves, chopped
lime zest

1. Peel grapefruit and oranges, then carefully cut out sections and squeeze any remaining juice into a bowl.
2. Add chopped mint and zest and any other fruit: sliced strawberries, blueberries, kiwi slices, diced mango. This looks especially pretty in a glass bowl.

Note: If you are taking statin drugs, replace the grapefruit with more oranges or other fruit.

Fruit, Fruit, Fruit with Ginger!

MAKES 8 SERVINGS

2 Asian pears, peeled and cut into bite-size pieces
1 pineapple, peeled, cored, and cut into bite-size pieces
1 mango, peeled and cut into bite-size pieces
1 box fresh raspberries
1 orange, peeled and sectioned, plus juice and zest
juice and zest of 1 lime
2 tablespoons peeled, grated fresh ginger

Combine all ingredients together and marvel at the flavor!

Roasted Pears with Maple Crunch

MAKES 4 SERVINGS

2 pears, halved lengthwise and seeded
2 teaspoons (or less) maple syrup
1/4 cup Grape-Nuts cereal

1. Preheat oven to 425 degrees.
2. Fill centers of pears with maple syrup, dividing evenly.
3. Put a small amount of water in bottom of a baking pan, add pear halves, and bake for 45 minutes.
4. Cover each pear half with Grape-Nuts, sprinkle with a little extra maple syrup, and bake a few minutes more.

Note: If you do not have heart disease, you can substitute toasted chopped walnuts for the Grape-Nuts.

Peaches Baked in Lemon and Ginger

MAKES 4 SERVINGS

1/3 cup (or less) sugar
1/4 cup fresh lemon juice
1 teaspoon peeled, grated fresh ginger, or 1/2 teaspoon ground ginger
2 tablespoons water
4 ripe peaches, halved and pitted
1 tablespoon Grape-Nuts cereal

1. Preheat oven to 425 degrees.
2. In a small saucepan, combine sugar, lemon juice, ginger, and water. Bring to a simmer.
3. Place peaches cut side up in a shallow 1-quart baking dish. Pour ginger syrup over peaches and into holes.
4. Bake for 15–20 minutes, or until peaches are tender when pierced with a knife and syrup has thickened.
5. Remove from oven, sprinkle on Grape-Nuts, and serve at room temperature. These are incredibly delicious and truly stand alone. For a special treat, try a dab of sorbet with them.

Note: If you do not have heart disease, you can substitute toasted walnuts for the Grape-Nuts.

Chocolate Mousse

MAKES 3–4 SERVINGS

Force yourself to make this serve three or four people. It is so good that it's not at all uncommon to find that just one person wants to eat it all!

1 12.3-ounce container light silken tofu, firm or extra firm
1/3 cup maple syrup, honey, or sugar
2 tablespoons unsweetened cocoa powder
1 teaspoon vanilla extract

Place all ingredients in a blender and process until smooth. Refrigerate or freeze 2 hours before serving. Serve in small bowls with little spoons and savor every bite.

VARIATIONS:

Add 1/4 teaspoon peppermint extract and garnish with a mint leaf. Or, blend 2 tablespoons raspberry syrup, 1 tablespoon honey, and 1/4 cup frozen raspberries and substitute for maple syrup.

Blueberry Purple Passion

MAKES 2–3 SERVINGS

1/2 cup light silken tofu
1 1/2 cups frozen blueberries (8–10 ounces)
2 tablespoons maple syrup, honey, agave nectar, or sugar
1 teaspoon vanilla extract

Place all ingredients in a blender and process until smooth. It may take a few minutes, but be patient: eventually the mixture will smooth out. This can be served immediately as a frozen dessert. Or you can wait until it thaws and serve it as a pudding—with fresh berries on top. If you triple the recipe, you can have it both ways: some frozen the first night and some pudding style the next (stir before serving as a pudding). Try adding a few drops of peppermint extract for variety.

Pineapple Paradise

MAKES 4 SERVINGS

This is a perfect light dessert and sweet enough to please any sweet tooth.

1 12.3-ounce container light extra-firm tofu
1 16-ounce can pineapple chunks, drained
1 tablespoon vanilla extract

Place all ingredients in a food processor or blender until well mixed. Serve in small bowls with small spoons. Possible toppings: dried pineapple, cherries, bananas, or raspberries, or toasted walnuts if you don't have heart disease.

Lemon Pie Parfait

MAKES 8 SERVINGS

After we saw the movie Million Dollar Baby, *I was determined to find a recipe for a "legal" lemon pie. Someone had sent Essy the* Lifestyle Center of America Cookbook, *and from it, I adapted both the lemon pie filling and the topping that follows. They are both quick and easy—and so good!*

2 cups pineapple juice
1/4 cup maple syrup, agave nectar, or honey
1/4 cup fresh lemon juice
7 tablespoons cornstarch or arrowroot
1 cup orange juice
1 tablespoon lemon zest

1. In a saucepan, stir together pineapple juice, maple syrup, and lemon juice. Bring to a boil.

2. Stir cornstarch into orange juice until mixture is smooth.
3. When pineapple juice reaches a boil, add orange juice mixture, stirring constantly. When it thickens—this happens quickly—it is done.
4. Remove from heat and add lemon zest.

VARIATIONS:

To make a lemon pie, pour mixture into a Grape-Nuts Piecrust (see recipe, page 282), top with Lemon Whipped Topping (see recipe below), and chill. To make a parfait, alternate layers of filling and topping (following recipe) in wineglasses or small bowls, and top with fresh berries.

Lemon Whipped Topping

1 12.3-ounce container light silken tofu, firm or extra-firm
2 tablespoons maple syrup
1 teaspoon vanilla extract
3 tablespoons fresh lemon juice
$\frac{1}{8}$ teaspoon lemon extract
fresh raspberries or blueberries

Place all ingredients in a blender and process until smooth. Chill. In addition to all the other recipes in which it plays a part, this topping is good on its own over blueberries or other fruit.

Birthday Cake

MAKES 8 SERVINGS

2 cups whole-wheat flour or barley flour

1 cup (or less) sugar

2 teaspoons baking powder

1 teaspoon baking soda

1 cup vanilla oat or nonfat soy milk

1 cup unsweetened applesauce

1 tablespoon vanilla extract

egg replacer for 2 eggs (2 tablespoons flaxseed meal mixed with 6 tablespoons water, or 1 tablespoon Ener-G egg replacer mixed with 4 tablespoons water)

1. Preheat oven to 350 degrees.
2. Mix first four ingredients in a medium bowl.
3. Mix remaining ingredients in a large bowl.
4. Pour dry ingredients into liquid and stir by hand or beat until no lumps remain.
5. Spread batter evenly between two 9-inch round cake pans or one 8 × 13-inch baking pan and bake for 35–40 minutes, until a toothpick inserted in center comes out clean and cake does not feel sticky when touched.
6. Cool before removing from pan. Serve plain, or top with fresh fruit, Pineapple Frosting, or Chocolate Sauce. For an amazing treat, frost with Lemon Pie Parfait topped with Lemon Whipped Topping. Even better, put some of the Lemon Pie Parfait between the 9-inch layers.

Carrot Cookie Cake

MAKES 6–8 SERVINGS

Our son-in-law, a teacher by trade but a chef at heart, suggested Grape-Nuts cereal to make the cake less moist. That did the trick!

1½ cups whole-wheat flour
½ cup Grape-Nuts cereal
1 teaspoon baking powder
¾ teaspoon baking soda
1 teaspoon ground cinnamon
½ cup maple syrup, honey, agave nectar, or brown sugar
egg replacer for 2 eggs (2 tablespoons flaxseed meal mixed with 6 tablespoons pineapple juice, or 1 tablespoon Ener-G egg replacer mixed with 4 tablespoons water)
1 cup shredded carrots
1 8-ounce can crushed pineapple, drained
¼ cup raisins (optional)
Pineapple Frosting (see below)
dried pineapple

1. Preheat oven to 350 degrees.
2. Mix first four ingredients well in a medium bowl.
3. Add remaining ingredients and mix. **Note:** If you have no heart disease, you might consider including ¼ cup chopped walnuts.
4. Scrape batter into two 9-inch round cake pans or one 9 × 13-inch pan and bake for 40 minutes, or until a toothpick inserted in center comes out clean. Cool completely.
5. Spread cooled cake with Pineapple Frosting (see below) and top with dried pineapple or fresh berries.

Note: This cake is very thin—but with frosting between layers and on top, it does look like a cake!

Pineapple Frosting

This is not sweet, and is unlike traditional frostings, but it is surprisingly good. This recipe makes enough to frost two cakes with leftovers. Try this on Carrot Cookie Cake or Chocolate Red Devil Cake.

1 12.3-ounce package light extra-firm tofu
1 16-ounce can pineapple chunks, drained (save the juice)
1/4 cup maple syrup, honey, agave nectar, or brown sugar
1/4 cup pineapple juice
2 tablespoons arrowroot
1 tablespoon vanilla extract
1/3 cup chopped dried pineapple (optional)

1. Place tofu in a food processor and process until smooth.
2. Add pineapple chunks, maple syrup, and pineapple juice and process until blended.
3. Add arrowroot and vanilla and blend.
4. Scrape into a saucepan and cook over medium-low heat for 5 minutes, stirring frequently. Cool.
5. Spread on cake and top with dried pineapple chunks.

Chocolate Red Devil Cake

MAKES 8–10 SERVINGS

For his fifth birthday, our grandson Zeb requested a chocolate cake. This recipe, adapted from Joanne Stepaniak's The Vegan Sourcebook, *sounded appealing. Zeb never had a clue he was eating beets!*

2 cups whole-wheat pastry flour or barley flour
1 cup sugar
1/2 cup unsweetened cocoa powder

2 teaspoons double-acting baking powder
2 teaspoons baking soda
2 tablespoons flaxseed meal
1/3 cup water
1 large beet, cooked and diced (1 cup)
1 cup water
1/3 cup baby-food prunes (1 large jar)
2 teaspoons apple-cider vinegar
2 teaspoons vanilla extract
Creamy Fudge Frosting (see below) or Pineapple Frosting (see page 278)

1. Preheat oven to 350 degrees. Use an 8-inch square baking pan, or two 9-inch round cake pans if you want icing between layers.
2. In a large mixing bowl, place flour, sugar, cocoa powder, baking powder, and baking soda and whisk until combined.
3. Place flaxseed meal in a dry blender. Add 1/3 cup water and blend about 30 seconds, until mixture is gummy. Add beets, water, prunes, vinegar, and vanilla and process 1–2 minutes, until frothy and well blended.
4. Mix liquid into dry ingredients. Stir until combined, then quickly spoon batter into pan.
5. Bake 35–40 minutes, until a toothpick inserted in the center comes out clean. Cool for at least 30 minutes. Spread cooled cake with Creamy Fudge Frosting or Pineapple Frosting.

Creamy Fudge Frosting

MAKES ENOUGH TO FROST A LAYER GENEROUSLY

1 12.3-ounce package light extra-firm tofu
1/3 cup maple syrup, agave nectar, or honey
2 tablespoons unsweetened cocoa powder
1 tablespoon vanilla extract

Combine all ingredients in food processor and process until smooth. Ice thickly on Chocolate Red Devil Cake. Even though it seems runny, the frosting stays on.

Luscious Lemon Cake

MAKES 6–8 SERVINGS

I adapted this cake from a recipe I got from Angie McIntosh, a wonderful plant-based cook who lives in Penticton, British Columbia. It is easy to make, very moist, and crazily good! We don't really know how it tastes after it cools because it never lasts long enough to find out.

egg replacer for 2 eggs (2 tablespoons flaxseed meal mixed with 6 tablespoons water, or 1 tablespoon Ener-G egg replacer mixed with 4 tablespoons water)
3/4 cup (or less) brown sugar
2 tablespoons fresh lemon juice
zest of 1 lemon
3/4 cup oat, almond, or nonfat soy milk
1/2 cup applesauce
2 teaspoons vanilla extract
1 1/2 cups whole-wheat flour
1 teaspoon baking soda
1 lemon half
granulated sugar

1. Preheat oven to 350 degrees.
2. Mix egg replacer and water in a large bowl. Add brown sugar, 2 tablespoons of lemon juice, lemon zest, milk, applesauce, and vanilla and stir well.
3. Mix flour and baking soda in a small bowl, then add to liquid and mix well.
4. Spoon into an 8-inch square baking pan and bake for 40 minutes, or until a toothpick inserted in center comes out clean.

5. Cool a little. Squeeze the juice from half a lemon (or more, if you like) over cake and sprinkle with granulated sugar.

Frozen Lemon Sorbet Cups

MAKES 6 SERVINGS

Our daughter-in-law, Anne Bingham, introduced us to these adorable and oh-so-easy dessert treats. Different sorbet colors on the top layer are fun. Try raspberry, mango, or blueberry. Children love to help and to choose their favorite flavor combinations.

1. Cut top inch off 6 large lemons and remove insides. Carefully shave bottoms off lemons so they will stand on their own.
2. Freeze lemons, including caps.
3. When frozen, fill each lemon to overflowing with sorbet of choice or a variety of flavors. Top with frozen lemon hat and refreeze until time to eat.

Raspberry Sorbet with Strawberry Sauce

MAKES 4 SERVINGS

I first ate this dessert at the Georgetown home of my aunt Kay Halle in Washington, D.C. Now we have it every Christmas Eve. It is beautiful and simple—everything can be prepared ahead of time—and everyone loves it! The most important thing to remember is that both the sorbet and the sauce should begin to melt before you serve the dessert.

1. Slightly thaw 1 pint raspberry sorbet, and spoon into a mold. (I use a heart-shaped mold, but anything will do. And since we usually have many people, I heap the heart with as many as 5 or 6 pints of sorbet.) Freeze mold.

2. When mold is frozen solid, dip into hot water or let stand until sorbet is soft enough to unmold into a bowl. Refreeze the sorbet in the bowl.
3. Slightly thaw one package of frozen light-sugar strawberry sauce (you can either let it stand at room temperature or place it in a bowl filled with water).
4. Put the partially frozen strawberry sauce in a food processor or blender and process until smooth. Refrigerate until using.
5. Thirty minutes before serving, remove sorbet from freezer. Pour most of strawberry sauce over sorbet. If a little is left, reserve in a pitcher. Put bowl in a warm place and allow sauce and sorbet to melt together.
6. Serve and pass the pitcher for a little extra sauce, if desired.
7. To repeat: this dessert is best when it softens and begins to run together. (Actually, we like it best when all the guests have gone, and there are only soft remainders of the sorbet remaining in the bowl!) Remove the sorbet from the freezer before guests sit down to dinner. Plan about 1 pint of sorbet to 1 package of frozen strawberries and as numbers increase, about 5 people to 1 pint of sorbet.

Grape-Nuts Piecrust

MAKES ONE 9-INCH CRUST

1–1¼ cups Grape-Nuts cereal, or enough to thinly cover the bottom of a pie plate

2–3 tablespoons frozen apple-juice concentrate (it spoons out quite easily)

1. Preheat oven to 350 degrees.
2. Pour Grape-Nuts into a 9-inch pie plate, add apple-juice concentrate, and mix until the cereal is moist but not wet.
3. Press Grape-Nuts up side of pie plate and bake for 10 minutes, until crust is nicely browned, watching constantly.

4. Cool crust in freezer or refrigerator until ready to fill.

Note: Fill at the last minute, so crust stays crisp.

Berry Pie Filling

MAKES ENOUGH FOR 1 PIE

1 quart fresh blueberries, strawberries, raspberries, or a mixture, sliced (or 1 16-ounce package of frozen berries)
1/3 cup frozen apple-juice concentrate
2 tablespoons cornstarch
1 banana (optional)

1. Put berries, apple-juice concentrate, and cornstarch into a saucepan and cook, stirring, over medium heat until mixture thickens.
2. Line Grape-Nuts Piecrust with sliced banana (optional). Cool berry mixture slightly and pour into piecrust. Serve immediately. (The crust gets soggy if it isn't eaten quickly—although it still tastes good.)

Very Easy Blueberry Cobbler

MAKES 4–6 SERVINGS

2/3 cup whole-wheat flour
1 1/2 teaspoons baking powder
2/3 cup oat, or nonfat soy milk
3 tablespoons maple syrup, sugar, or honey
1 tablespoon vanilla extract
2 cups blueberries

1. Preheat oven to 350 degrees.
2. Combine flour and baking powder in a small bowl.
3. Combine milk, maple syrup, and vanilla in a measuring cup and stir, then add to flour and mix until smooth. (Batter will be quite runny.)
4. Pour batter into a nonstick 8-inch square pan. Sprinkle berries on top.
5. Bake for 45 minutes, or until lightly browned. A few tablespoons of any sorbet are delicious with this.

Mixed Berry Cobbler

MAKES 9 SERVINGS

BERRY MIXTURE:

6 cups fresh or frozen berries (boysenberries, blackberries, raspberries, or a mixture)

3 tablespoons whole-wheat flour or barley flour

1/4 cup sugar, maple syrup, agave nectar, or honey

TOPPING:

1 cup whole-wheat flour or barley flour

2 tablespoons sugar or maple syrup

1 1/2 teaspoons baking powder

2/3 cup oat, almond, or nonfat soy milk

2 teaspoons vanilla extract

1. Preheat oven to 375 degrees.
2. Spread berries in a 9-inch square nonstick baking dish and mix in flour and sugar.
3. Bake about 15 minutes, until hot.
4. While berries are heating, prepare topping: mix flour, sugar, and baking powder. (If using maple syrup, add that in next step.)
5. Mix milk and vanilla together and stir into batter until it is smooth.

6. Spread batter evenly over hot berries (don't worry if they are not completely covered), then bake for 25–30 minutes, until golden brown. A dab of any sorbet is good with this.

Chewy Gingerbread Cookies

MAKES 2 DOZEN SMALL COOKIES

This is adapted from one of Martha Stewart's most popular cookie recipes. With whole-wheat flour, no semisweet chocolate, and no butter, it is still good. Our four-year-old granddaughter, Bainon, loved making the balls and rolling them in sugar. We were too impatient to put the dough in the refrigerator, so she was covered from wrist to fingertips with sticky dough—part of the fun! If you are in a hurry, just spoon out the dough and sprinkle with a little sugar, if desired.

1½ cups whole-wheat pastry flour or barley flour
2 tablespoons unsweetened cocoa powder
1¼ teaspoons ground ginger
1 teaspoon ground cinnamon
¼ teaspoon ground cloves
¼ teaspoon ground nutmeg
½ cup baby-food prunes or applesauce
1 tablespoon peeled, finely chopped fresh ginger
½ cup packed brown sugar
¼ cup unsulphered molasses
1 teaspoon baking soda dissolved in 1¼ teaspoons boiling water
¼ cup granulated sugar

1. Preheat oven to 325 degrees.
2. Put flour, cocoa, and spices into a medium bowl and set aside.
3. Put prunes and ginger into bowl of electric mixer and blend on medium speed until well mixed. Add brown sugar; mix until combined. Add molasses; mix until combined.

4. Add flour mixture in 2 batches, alternating with baking soda mixture.
5. Dissolve baking soda in boiling water.
6. Transfer dough to a piece of plastic wrap and pat to a 1-inch thickness. Refrigerate until firm, or until you can't wait any longer (if you don't wait, the dough will be really sticky)!
7. Line 2 baking sheets with parchment paper. Roll dough into 1 1/2-inch balls, then roll balls in granulated sugar. Space balls 2 inches apart on prepared baking sheets.
8. Bake for 20 minutes, or until surfaces crack slightly. Cool on sheets for 5 minutes. Transfer to a wire rack and cool completely.

Note: To make cupcakes, increase applesauce or prunes to 1 cup, put dough in small cupcake tins and bake as above.

Oatmeal-Maple Cookies

MAKES ABOUT 1 DOZEN COOKIES IF YOU USE 1/2 CUP RAISINS

1 cup oats
2/3 cup oat bran
2 tablespoons flaxseed meal
1/3–1/2 cup raisins
1/3 cup maple syrup, brown sugar, agave nectar, or honey
1/2 cup oat milk or water
1 tablespoon vanilla extract

1. Preheat oven to 350 degrees.
2. Toast oats until golden brown. Watch carefully so they don't burn.
3. While oats are toasting, put remaining ingredients in the above order in a medium bowl. Add toasted oats and mix well.
4. Put 10–12 tablespoons of dough on a nonstick baking sheet and flatten with the back of a fork.
5. Bake for 25 minutes, or until slightly golden on edges. Check often to prevent burning.

Acknowledgments

The scope and depth of this project could never have been achieved without the help of many to whom I would like to express my thanks.

First, a special tribute to my late brother-in-law George Crile III and his wife, Susan Lyne. From the start, George—a marvelously talented journalist, television producer, and author—was inspired by the research and fascinated by the human dimension of my patients' recovery. Although he refused to sign his name to it, he is responsible for the compelling introduction to this book.

My secretary Irene Greenberg was also an early and enthusiastic supporter of the project. After Irene's untimely death in 1988, Sandy Gobozy took over the secretarial duties and patiently retyped draft after draft of my manuscript while helping to nurture our patients.

The following Cleveland Clinic cardiologists referred patients for the research: doctors Stephan Ellis, Irving Franco, Jay Holman, Frederick Pashkow, Russ Raymond, Ernest Salcedo, William Sheldon, Earl Shirey, and Donald Underwood. Particular thanks to cardiologist James Hodgman, for reviewing the manuscript, and Bernadine Healy, who in 1985, at the inception of my research, offered guidance and wisdom.

Kindred spirits in the transition to healthier living have my gratitude for their own inspiring work. Among them: Neal Barnard, Colin Campbell, Antonia Demas, Hans Diehl, Joel Fuhrman, Mladen Galubic, Alan Goldhammer, William Harris, Michael Jacobson, Michael Klaper, Robert Kradjian, Doug Lisle, Howard Lyman, John McDougall, Jeff Nelson, Dean Ornish, and John Robbins.

Tim Crowe, a brilliant imaging technician in the Cleveland Clinic angiography core laboratory, was responsible for the accurate and powerful angiogram findings that are reported and reproduced in this book. And the reperfusion research would have been impossible without the help of doctors Richard Brunken, Raymondo Go, and Kandice Marchant.

Cleveland Clinic chief executive officers, William Kaiser and Floyd Loop, and my department chairman, Robert Hermann, graciously allowed me one half day a week away from my surgical duties to do my research.

Abraham Brickner, a colleague, friend, and patient, offered helpful criticism along with unyielding belief in my nutrition-based approach to preventing and reversing heart disease.

Julia Brandi provided invaluable assistance in setting up the First National Conference on the Prevention and Elimination of Coronary Artery Disease, where my research first made its mark.

I owe particular thanks to Dr. Joe Crowe and his wife, Mary Lind, whose one hundred percent commitment to my program produced some of the most spectacular proof so far that heart disease can be reversed. The remarkable angiograms showing Dr. Crowe's progress have inspired many others to try our approach.

My late sister, Dr. Sally Esselstyn Howell, her husband, Dr. Rodney Howell, and my brother Erik Esselstyn all have provided unwavering support through the years.

My late father, Caldwell B. Esselstyn, M.D., has always been an inspiration. He taught me that you must never quit when you know you are right. And long before it became fashionable, he argued that the only way out of the impossible health-care burden that confronts the United States is to teach people how to live healthier lives.

My children, Rip, Ted, Jane, and Zeb; their spouses, Anne Bingham, Brian Hart, and Jill Kolasinski; and my grandchildren, Flinn Esselstyn, Gus Esselstyn, Rose Esselstyn, Crile Hart, Zeb Hart, and Bainon Hart, all have embraced plant-based eating. I am grateful to every one of them, and cherish all the fun we have sharing meals. Special thanks to my son Ted for the endothelial drawing and for the delightful vegetable illustrations in the recipe section of this book.

I enthusiastically thank the Avery group at Penguin—publisher Megan Newman and her team, Lucia Watson, Kate Stark, and Lissa Brown—whose skills, insights, and expertise have been essential in developing this book.

My agent, Peter Bernstein, has been a source of wisdom, guidance, and friendship. I am especially indebted to him for finding my gifted collaborator, Merrill McLoughlin. Mimi has helped make my biological research understandable and accessible, weaving into the hard science the very human stories of my original patients. The result, I think, is a book that will educate and bring hope to many.

Finally, I am forever obligated to my wife, Ann, for her unflinching loyalty when resistance to my ideas and research seemed insurmountable. She encouraged, helped rewrite, and constantly renewed my belief in myself and my commitment to the passion that was driving me. Working like a Trojan for more than twenty-two years, she has developed, modified, and tested all the plant-based recipes at the end of this book. It is dedicated to her.

Notes

1. Eating to Live

1. Government Accountability Office.
2. Lewis H. Kuller, et al., *Archives of Internal Medicine*, January 9, 2006: "10-year Follow-up of Subclinical Cardiovascular Disease and Risk of Coronary Heart Disease in the Cardiovascular Health Study."
3. Bertram Pitt, David Waters, et al., *New England Journal of Medicine*, July 8, 1999: "Aggressive Lipid-lowering Therapy Compared with Angioplasty in Stable Coronary Artery Disease."

2. "Someday We'll Have to Get Smarter"

1. G. Bjerregarrd and A. Jung'u, *East African Medical Journal*, January 1991: "Breast Cancer in Kenya: A Histopathologic and Epidemiologic Study."
2. K. M. Dalessandri and C. H. Organ Jr., *American Journal of Surgery*, April 1995: "Surgery, Drugs, Lifestyle and Hyperlipidemia."
3. T. Colin Campbell with Thomas M. Campbell II, *The China Study*, BenBella Books, 2005.
4. National Heart, Lung and Blood Institute, National Institutes of Health.
5. R. W. Wissler, D. Vesselinovitch, *Advanced Veterinary Science Comp Med*, 1977: "Atherosclerosis in Nonhuman Primates."

3. Seeking the Cure

1. Campbell with Campbell.
2. The most frequent dosage was 4 grams, twice a day, of cholestyramine, and 40 to 60 milligrams daily of lovastatin.

4. A Primer on Heart Disease

1. K. M. Dalessandri and C. H. Organ, Jr., *American Journal of Surgery*, April 1995: "Surgery, Drugs, Lifestyle and Hyperlipidemia."
2. Campbell with Campbell.
3. W. Castelli, J. Doyle, T. Gordon, et al., *Circulation*, May 1977: "HDL Cholesterol and Other Lipids in Coronary Heart Disease."

5. Moderation Kills

1. N. B. Oldridge, G. H. Guyatt, M. E. Fischer, and A. A. Rimm, *Journal of the American Medical Association*, August 19, 1988: "Cardiac Rehabilitation After Myocardial Infarction; Combined Experience of Randomized Clinical Trials."
2. Various authors, *Journal of the American Medical Association*, February 8, 2006: "Low-Fat Dietary Pattern and Risk of Invasive Breast Cancer"; "Low-Fat Dietary Pattern and Risk of Colorectal Cancer and Low-Fat Dietary Pattern and Risk of Cardiovascular Disease: The Women's Health Initiative Randomized Controlled Dietary Modification Trial."

3. W. C. Roberts, *American Journal of Cardiology,* September 1, 1989: "Atherosclerotic Risk Factors—Are There Ten or Is There Only One?"
4. R. Luyken, F. Luyken-Louing, and N. Pikaar, *American Journal of Clinical Nutrition,* 1964: "Nutrition Studies in New Guinea; Epidemiological Studies in a Highland Population of New Guinea: Environment, Culture and Health Status."
5. N. Werner, et al., *New England Journal of Medicine,* September 8, 2005: "Circulating Endothelial Progenitor Cells and Cardiovascular Outcomes."
6. Robert A. Vogel, *Clinical Cardiology,* June 1999: "Brachial Artery Ultrasound: A Noninvasive Tool in the Assessment of Triglyceride-Rich Lipoproteins."
7. Christopher P. Cannon, et al., *New England Journal of Medicine,* April 8, 2004: "Intensive versus Moderate Lipid Lowering with Statins After Acute Coronary Syndromes."
8. The Nobel laureates: Drs. Robert F. Furchgott, Ferid Murad, and Louis J. Ignarro.

6. Living, Breathing Proof

1. E. A. Brinton, S. Eisenberg, and J. L. Breslow, *Journal of Clinical Investigation,* January 1990: "A Low-fat Diet Decreases High-Density Lipoprotein (HDL) Cholesterol Levels by Decreasing HDL Apolipoprotein Transport Rates."

7. Why Didn't Anyone Tell Me?

1. K. L. Gould, *Circulation,* September 1994: "Reversal of Coronary Atherosclerosis: Clinical Promise as the Basis for Noninvasive Management of Coronary Artery Disease."
2. J. Stamler, D. Wentworth, and J. D. Neaton, for MRFIT Research Group, *Journal of the American Medical Association,* November 28, 1986: "Is Relationship Between Serum Cholesterol and Risk of Premature Death from Coronary Heart Disease Continuous and Graded?"
3. W. Castelli, *Prevention,* November 1996: "Take This Letter to Your Doctor."
4. *Nutrition Action,* September 2004, Volume 31.
5. Campbell with Campbell.
6. T. Colin Campbell, from an address to the First National Conference for the Elimination of Coronary Artery Disease, October 1991, Tucson, AZ; quoted by Charles Attwood, M.D., in an interview with the author.
7. Increasing interest in coronary disease prevention led to the 2nd National Conference on Lipids in the Elimination and Prevention of Coronary Artery Disease, held in association with The Disney Company in Orlando, Florida, in September 1997. The theme: shifting the paradigm of treatment from invasive symptomatic treatments toward arrest and reversal of disease through nutritional changes. The proceedings were published as a supplement to the *American Journal of Cardiology,* November 26, 1998.

8. Simple Steps

1. D. J. Jenkins, et al., *New England Journal of Medicine,* October 5, 1989: "Nibbling versus Gorging: Metabolic Advantages of Increased Meal Frequency."

9. Frequently Asked Questions

1. R. D. Mattes, *American Journal of Clinical Nutrition,* March 1993: "Fat Preference and Adherence to a Reduced-fat Diet."
2. M. H. Frick, et al., *New England Journal of Medicine,* November 12, 1987: "Helsinki Heart Study: Primary-prevention Trial with Gemfibrozil in Middle-aged Men with Dyslipidemia. Safety of Treatment, Changes in Risk Factors and Incidence of Coronary Heart Disease."
3. G. Weidner, S. L. Connor, J. F. Hollis, and W. E. Connor, *Annals of Internal Medicine,* 1992: "Improvements in Hostility and Depression in Relation to Dietary Change and Cholesterol Lowering. The Family Heart Study."
4. *The Lancet,* November 19, 1994, Scandinavian Simvastatin Survival Study Group: "Randomized Trial of Cholesterol Lowering in 4,444 Patients with Coronary Heart Disease."

10. Why Can't I Have "Heart Healthy" Oils?

1. Michel de Lorgeril, et al., *Circulation,* February 16, 1999: "Mediterranean Diet, Traditional Risk Factors, and the Rate of Cardiovascular Complications After Myocardial Infarction; Final Report of the Lyon Diet Heart Study."
2. D. H. Blankenhorn, R. Johnson, et al., *Journal of the American Medical Association,* March 23, 1990: "The Influence of Diet on the Appearance of New Lesions in Human Coronary Arteries."
3. Lawrence L. Rudel, John S. Parks, and Janet K. Sawyer, *Arteriosclerosis, Thrombosis, and Vascular Biology,* December 1995: "Compared with Dietary Monounsaturated and Saturated Fat, Polyunsaturated Fat Protects African Green Monkeys from Coronary Artery Arteriosclerosis."
4. R. Vogel, M. Corretti, and G. Plotnick, *Journal of the American College of Cardiology,* 2000: "The Postprandial Effect of Compo-

nents of the Mediterranean Diet on Endothelial Function."

5. N. Tsunoda, S. Ikemoto, M. Takahashi, et al., *Metabolism,* June 1998: "High Monounsaturated Fat Diet-induced Obesity and Diabetes."

11. Kindred Spirits

1. J. D. Hubbard, S. Inkeles, and R. J. Barnard, *New England Journal of Medicine,* July 4, 1985: "Nathan Pritikin's Heart."
2. Steven Aldana, Roger Greenlaw, Hans Diehl, Audrey Salberg, Ray Merrill, Seiga Ohime, and Camille Thomas, *Journal of the American Dietetic Association* 105 (2005): "Effects of an Intensive Diet and Physical Activity Modification Program on the Health Risks of Adults." Heike Englert, Hans Diehl, and Roger Greenlaw, *Preventive Medicine* 38 (2004): "Rationale and Design of the Rockford CHIP, a Community-Based Coronary Risk Reduction Program: Results of a Pilot Phase."
3. Viking, 352 pages.

12. Brave New World

1. National Center for Health Statistics, Centers for Disease Control and Prevention.
2. Pierre Aramenco et al., *New England Journal of Medicine,* December 1, 1994: "Atherosclerotic Disease of the Aortic Arch and the Risk of Ischemic Stroke."
3. Mark F. Newman et al., *New England Journal of Medicine,* February 8, 2001: "Longitudinal Assessment of Neurocognitive Function after Coronary Artery Bypass Surgery."
4. Sarah E. Vermeer et al., *New England Journal of Medicine,* March 27, 2003: "Silent Brain Infarcts and the Risk of Dementia and Cognitive Decline."
5. Ingmar Skoog et al., *New England Journal of Medicine,* January 21, 1993: "A Population Study of Dementia in 85-year-olds."
6. M. Breteler et al., *British Medical Journal,* June 18, 1994: "Cardiovascular Disease and Distribution of Cognitive Function in Elderly People—The Rotterdam Study."
7. Ian M. Thompson, et al., *Journal of the American Medical Association,* December 21, 2005: "Erectile Dysfunction and Subsequent Cardiovascular Disease."
8. James Fries and Lawrence Crapo, *Vitality and Aging,* W. H. Freeman & Co., 1981.

13. You Are in Control

1. René G. Favaloro, *Journal of the American College of Cardiology,* March 15, 1998: "Critical Analysis of Coronary Artery Bypass Graft Surgery: a 30-Year Journey."
2. John P. Cooke and Judith Zimmer, *The Cardiovascular Cure: How to Strengthen Your Self-Defense Against Heart Attack and Stroke,* Broadway, 2002.
3. James S. Forrester and Prediman K. Shah, *Circulation,* August 19, 1997: "Lipid Lowering Versus Revascularization: An Idea Whose Time (for Testing) Has Come."
4. Demosthenes D. Katritsis and John Ioannidis, *Circulation,* June 7, 2005: "Percutaneous Coronary Intervention Versus Conservative Therapy in Nonacute Coronary Artery Disease."
5. The Cleveland Clinic Heart Advisor, June 2006: "What to Do About Chest Pain: Your Knowledgeable Response to Discomfort Could Save Your Life."

14. Simple Strategies

1. R. D. Mattes, *American Journal of Clinical Nutrition,* March 1993: "Fat Preference and Adherence to a Reduced-fat Diet."

Appendix I

Safe Food

Below is a list of some of the plant-based products we have found that are made from 100% whole grain and contain no oil and lower levels of sodium and sugar. Some are widely available in ordinary supermarkets; others can be found only in health food stores (for example, Trader Joe's and Wild Oats brands are sold primarily through their own outlets). See Appendix III for help in finding products your local stores don't carry.

Remember, products change constantly. ALWAYS read labels. Don't trust that because one loaf of bread made by a company is "safe," all of its bread will be.

BREAD

Aladdin's pocket pita bread
Alvarado Street Bakery bagels and buns
Ezekiel 4:9 sprouted grain breads, buns, and tortillas
French Meadow spelt, rye, and whole-grain
Genuine Bavarian Bread whole-grain, flaxseed, multigrain, and sunflower-seed
Great Harvest Bread Company (Be sure to check labels.)
Lahvash fat-free authentic wraps
Mestemacher pumpernickel, whole-rye, flaxseed, and three-grain breads
Paramount whole-wheat lavash
Reinecker's Bolkorn Brot
Trader Joe's whole-wheat pita bread
Wild Oats organic tortillas (whole-wheat, yellow corn)
Wild Oats yellow corn organic tortillas

BROTH

Health Valley fat-free vegetable broth (360 mg sodium)
Kitchen Basics roasted vegetable stock (330 mg sodium)
Pacific Organic fat-free vegetable broth and fat-free mushroom broth (530 mg sodium)
Pacific Organic low-sodium vegetable broth (140 mg sodium)
Trader Joe's fat-free organic vegetable broth (330 mg sodium)

CEREAL

Barbara's Bakery shredded wheat (no-sugar)
Erewhon raisin bran
Grainfield's whole-grain raisin bran and multigrain flakes cereals
Grape-Nuts
Post shredded wheat and bran
Shredded wheat
Trader Joe's shredded bite-size wheats

CHIPS

Guiltless Gourmet baked unsalted yellow corn chips (the only oil-free chips Guiltless Gourmet makes)
Frito-Lay's Tostitos baked corn chips

COOKIES/SWEETS

Barbara's Wheat-free fig bars (Avoid raspberry, with added glycerin, and whole-wheat, with canola oil.)
Just Bananas dried fruits and vegetables

CRACKERS

Edward & Sons brown rice snaps (tamari-sesame, onion-garlic, and unsalted)
Hol-Grain crackers (no-salt and brown rice)
Ryvita (sesame rye, etc.)
San-J tamari brown rice crackers (Don't confuse with the sesame tamari brown rice crackers.)
Wasa Original Crispbread (Read ingredients: some contain mono- and diglycerides.)
Kavli Crispy Thin crispbread
Scandinavian Bran Crispbread (Sesame only; toasted onion and vegetable contain safflower oil—avoid them.)
Wheat Weavers (from Wild Oats and Whole Foods)

HOT DOGS/VEGGIE BURGERS/CHILI

Health Valley 99% fat-free vegetarian chili, mild black bean chili, spicy black bean chili, and mild three-bean chili
Lightlife Smart Dogs
Vegan Burger (Price Chopper)
Whole Foods organic vegan veggie burger
Yves Veggie Cuisine Veggie Dogs

HUMMUS/SPREADS/DIPS

Guiltless Gourmet mild black bean dip
Oasis Classic Cuisine zero-fat hummus, Mediterranean medley, shiitake mushroom, and roasted red pepper (all without tahini)
Sahara Cuisine black bean and lentil dips
Sahara Cuisine original hummus and organic roasted red pepper (both without tahini)
Trader Joe's mango salsa and pineapple salsa

ICE CREAM/SORBET

Dole sorbet in fruit flavors (Beware: Dole's chocolate sorbet contains egg whites.)
Dreyer's whole-fruit bars
Edy's whole-fruit products (bars, sorbets)
Häagen-Dazs sorbet
Sweet Nothings nondairy fudge bar and mango-raspberry bar

PASTA

Ancient Harvest quinoa
Bionature organic pasta—penne, fusilli, and rigatoni pastas
DeBoles whole-wheat spaghetti-style pasta, penne, and angel hair pastas
Eden Organic traditionally made udon, soba, spelt, and brown-rice pastas
Hodgson Mill whole-wheat lasagna and elbows
Lindburg brown-rice pasta, rotini, and penne
Tinkyada brown-rice pasta, spirals, penne, shells, fettuccine, and lasagne
VitaSpelt whole-grain pasta, elbows, and rotini
Wild Oats whole-wheat fusilli, kamut, spaghetti, and spelt

PASTA SAUCE

Muir Glen mushroom marinara and portobello mushroom pasta sauces
Trader Joe's organic spaghetti sauce with mushrooms
Walnut Acres low-sodium Tomato Basil Pasta Sauce
Whole Foods' 365 Organic Pasta Sauce

PIZZA CRUST

Nature's Hilights brown-rice pizza crust

POLENTA/MOCHI

Grainaissance mochi—original, pizza, raisin-cinnamon, sesame-garlic, mugwort-wheatgrass
Monterey Pasta Company, Nate's 100% organic polenta
Trader Joe's organic polenta

TOFU/SEITAN

Lightlife organic seitan
Mori-Nu light low-fat silken tofu (extra-firm, firm, soft)
White Wave seitan

Appendix II

Resources

USEFUL COOKBOOKS

The following list represents a selection of books that have been helpful to us. You will find others as you begin to look yourself. Please note that recipes in some books must be altered in order to meet your needs, whatever they might be: no salt, no sugar, and no nuts, for instance. Just follow the rules. Always look for plant-based recipes, whole grains and, of course, *no oil*. The best advice we can offer about cookbook recipes is the same we stress when it comes to packaged foods: *Read the ingredients*. You can almost always adapt a recipe so that it meets your standards for safe eating.

The Accidental Vegan, by Devra Gartenstein, Crossing Press, 2000. A little book with good recipes that contain no meat, fish, poultry, or dairy products.

The (Almost) No-Fat Cookbook: Everyday Vegetarian Recipes and *The (Almost) No-Fat Holiday Cookbook: Festive Vegetarian Recipes,* by Bryanna Clark Grogan, Book Publishing Company, 1994 and 1995, respectively. Creative and appealing recipes containing no meat, fish, poultry, dairy products, or oil.

CalciYum! Delicious Calcium-Rich Dairy-Free Vegetarian Recipes, by David and Rachelle Bronfman, Bromedia, Inc., 1998. Very good calcium-rich recipes with no meat, fish, poultry, or dairy products. Avoid the recipes that contain oil and nuts.

The Candle Café Cookbook, by Joy Pierson and Bart Potenza with Barbara Scott-Goodman, Clarkson Potter, 2003. Based on cooking at the New York restaurant of the same name, this contains wonderful vegan recipes, a few of which can be adapted to no-fat eating.

Dr. Attwood's Low-Fat Prescription for Kids, by Charles R. Attwood, M.D., Viking, 1995. An excellent book for children—and the whole family—it includes recipes that contain no meat, fish, poultry, or dairy products, but some oil.

Eat More, Weigh Less, by Dean Ornish, M.D., HarperCollins, 2001, and *Everyday Cooking with Dr. Dean Ornish,* HarperCollins, 1997. These books have delicious recipes with no meat, fish, poultry, or oil, and it is easy to use nondairy substitutes.

Eat to Live: The Revolutionary Formula for Fast and Sustained Weight Loss, by Joel Fuhrman, M.D., Little, Brown and Company, 2003. Also see Dr. Fuhrman's *Disease-Proof Your*

Child, St. Martin's Press, 2005. These books—containing no meat, fish, poultry, dairy products, or oil in the ingredients—are excellent for truly nutrient-dense recipes.

Fat Free and Delicious, by Robert N. Siegel, Pacifica Press, 1996. One of my favorites. Its delicious and varied recipes contain no meat, fish, poultry, dairy products, or oil.

Fat-Free & Easy: Great Meals in Minutes, by Jennifer Raymond, Book Publishing Company, 1997. Another book with fabulous plant-based, no-oil recipes. Jennifer Raymond makes it truly easy to eat this way!

The Health Promoting Cookbook: Simple, Guilt-Free, Vegetarian Recipes, by Alan Goldhamer, Book Publishing Company, 1997. An outstanding collection of basic recipes for health without meat, fish, poultry, dairy products, or oil.

Life Tastes Better Than Steak: Cookbook, by Gerry Krag and Marie Zimolzak, Avery Color Studios, 1996. No meat, fish, poultry, or oil is used. Avoid recipes that call for low-fat dairy products and egg whites.

The McDougall Quick & Easy Cookbook, by John A. McDougall, M.D., and Mary McDougall, Plume, 1999; *The New McDougall Cookbook,* Plume, 1997; *The McDougall Program for Maximum Weight Loss,* Plume, 1995. All the McDougall cookbooks are outstanding, with recipes for every occasion and every taste. They are the first we recommend to people who are changing their eating, and our holiday meals are always based on Mary McDougall's recipes.

The Millennium Cookbook: Extraordinary Vegetarian Cuisine, by Eric Tucker and John Westerdahl with dessert recipes by Sascha Weiss, Ten Speed Press, 1998. The Millennium Restaurant in San Francisco is one of the best vegan restaurants in the world. These recipes are often high in fat, but some can be easily adapted.

The Moosewood Cookbook, by Mollie Katzen, Ten Speed Press, 2000 (revised edition). This cookbook and its many sequels introduced many Americans to vegetarian cooking. Avoid the dairy products and oil.

The RAVE Diet & Lifestyle, by Mike Anderson, Beacon DV, 2004. No meat, fish, poultry, dairy products, or oil. Filled with good, safe recipes (www.ravediet.com).

The Taste for Living Cookbook: Mike Milken's Favorite Recipes for Fighting Cancer, by Beth Ginsberg and Michael Milken, CaP Cure, 1998. Creative and delicious recipes without meat, fish, poultry, dairy products, or oil. Avoid the processed soy and egg whites, no matter how tempting the pictures make them seem!

The Vegan Sourcebook, by Joanne Stepaniak, McGraw-Hill, 2000. There's no meat, fish, poultry, or dairy products in this comprehensive book. But beware of oil and nuts.

Vegetarian Cooking with Jeanie Burke, R.D., by Jeanie Burke, self-published, 2003 (available through her website, www.jeanieskitchen.com). Some good ideas, with no meat, poultry, or fish. But avoid the dairy products, oil, and nuts.

A Vegetarian's Ecstasy, by James Levin, M.D., and Natalie Cederquist, GLO Publishing, 1994. Delicious recipes with no meat, fish, poultry, or dairy products and very little oil.

Additional Reading: The titles below are not strictly recipe books, but we highly recommend them for anyone interested in good health:

The China Study, by T. Colin Campbell with Thomas M. Campbell II, BenBella Books, 2005. If you have any doubts about a plant-based diet, this book will turn you into a plant-based warrior! It should be required reading for everyone.

Turn Off the Fat Genes, Three Rivers Press, 2001, and *Breaking the Food Seduction: The Hidden Reasons Behind Food Cravings—and 7 Steps to End Them Naturally,* by Neal Barnard, M.D., St. Martin's Press, 2003. These books contain some recipes (beware of the oil in *Breaking the Food Seduction*), but the main point is their important message.

No More Bull!: The Mad Cowboy Targets America's Worst Enemy: Our Diet, by Howard F. Lyman, Glen Merzer, and Joanna Samorow-Merzer, Scribner, 2005. A powerful argument for plant-based eating. It includes recipes; just leave out the oil in some.

The Pleasure Trap: Mastering the Hidden Force that Undermines Health & Happiness, by Douglas J. Lisle and Alan Goldhamer, Healthy Living Publications, 2003. The authors propose a solution to man's basic physiologic drives, which are responsible for prevailing chronic illness.

Becoming Vegan: The Complete Guide to Adopting a Healthy Plant-Based Diet, by Brenda Davis and Vesanto Melina, Book Publishing Company, 2000. Good advice from real pros.

Food Is Elementary: A Hands-on Curriculum for Young Students, by Antonia Demas, Food Studies Institute, 2001. Twenty-eight lesson plans about healthy eating for kids by a plant-based chef who is working to change the lunches served in American schools.

Health Power, by Aileen Ludington and Hans Diehl. Review & Herald Publishing Association, 2000. This user-friendly book is full of information to prevent and reverse many killer diseases.

HELPFUL WEBSITES

The sites listed below contain all sorts of helpful advice and recipes. One in particular—www.engine2.org—has special meaning for us. It is the website of a group of firefighters at Fire Station No. 2 in Austin, Texas, who have dedicated themselves to healthy eating. Our son Rip is one of them. Their motto: "Fight fire, fight cholesterol, fight fat."

www.drmcdougall.com—an excellent free monthly newsletter, plus safe recipes
www.vegdining.com—a guide to vegetarian restaurants around the world
www.fatfree.com—fat-free recipes (but be vigilant about oil, dairy products, and white flour)
www.grainaissance.com—organic brown-rice products and recipes
www.ivu.org—vegetarian recipes with an international flair (but be careful about oil)
www.veganculinaryexperience.com
www.vegparadise.com—wonderful suggestions for products and recipes
www.vegsource.com—the largest, most trafficked vegetarian website on the Internet
www.engine2.org—Rip's team of fire- and fat-fighters

MANUFACTURERS AND PRODUCTS

This is by no means an exhaustive list, but it may help you find products you need.

ALVARADO STREET BAKERY—Organic sprouted whole-grain breads, buns, and bagels
500 Martin Ave.
Rohnert Park, CA 94928
www.alvaradostreetbakery.com
707-585-3293
Fax: 707-585-8954

ARROWHEAD MILLS—Whole-grain products and cereals
The Hain Celestial Group
4600 Sleepytime Drive
Boulder, CO 80301
www.arrowheadmills.com
1-800-434-4246

Bob's Red Mill Natural Foods—Whole-grain products and ground flaxseed
5209 SE International Way
Milwaukie, OR 97222
www.bobsredmill.com
1-800-349-2173
Fax: 503-653-1339

DeBoles—Organic and whole-wheat pastas
The Hain Celestial Group
4600 Sleepytime Dr.
Boulder, CO 80301
www.deboles.com
1-800-434-4246

Food for Life Baking Co., Inc.—Organic, flourless products, including Ezekiel 4:9 sprouted breads, buns, and tortillas
PO Box 1434
Corona, CA 92878
www.foodforlife.com
1-800-797-5090

Great Harvest Bread Company—Whole-grain breads (but double-check ingredients)
28 S. Montana St.
Dillon, MT 59725
www.greatharvest.com
1-800-442-0424 or 406-683-6842
Fax: 406-683-5537

Guiltless Gourmet—Dips, unsalted no-oil corn chips (other GG chips contain oil)
R.A.B. Food Group, LLC
One Harmon Plaza, 10th Floor
Secaucus, NJ 07094
www.guiltlessgourmet.com

Health Valley—Soups, broths, and fat-free meal cups
The Hain Celestial Group
4600 Sleepytime Dr.
Boulder, CO 80301
www.healthvalley.com
1-800-434-4246

Hodgson Mill—Whole-grain flours, cereals, and pastas; online catalog
1100 Stevens Ave.
Effingham, IL 62401
www.hodgsonmill.com
1-800-347-0105
Fax: 217-347-0198

Hudson Valley Homestead—Condiments galore, especially mustards
102 Sheldon La.
Craryville, NY 12521
www.hudsonvalleyhomestead.com
518-851-7336
Fax: 518-851-7553

Just Tomatoes, etc.—Dried fruits and vegetables
PO Box 807
Westley, CA 95387
www.justtomatoes.com
1-800-537-1985 (orders) or 209-894-5371
Fax: 1-800-537-1986 (orders) or 209-894-3146

Kitchen Basics—Roasted vegetable stock; recipes
PO Box 41022
Brecksville, OH 44141
www.kitchenbasics.net
440-838-1344

Mestemacher—Whole-grain breads and cereals from Germany
Am Anger 16
D-33332 Gütersloh
Postfach 2451 D-33254
Germany
www.germandeli.com/mebr.html

Muir Glen—Two no-oil pasta sauces (mushroom marinara and portobello mushroom)
Small Planet Foods
PO Box 9452
Minneapolis, MN 55440
www.muirglen.com
1-800-624-4123

Natural Market Place—Brown-rice pizza crust, Bragg Liquid Aminos
4719 Lower Roswell Rd.
Marietta, GA 30068
www.naturalmarketplace.net
770-973-4061

Nature's Path Foods—Pastas, cereals, Manna Bread (a cake-like sprouted-grain bread with no oil, sweeteners, or salt; comes in several flavors—delicious, toasted)
9100 Van Horne Way
Richmond, BC
V6X 1W3
Canada
www.naturespath.com
1-888-808-9505

Oasis Mediterranean Cuisine—Hummus without tahini
1520 Laskey Rd.
Toledo, OH 43612
419-269-1459

Pacific Foods—Fat-free vegetable and mushroom broths
19480 SW 97th Ave.
Tualatin, OR 97062
www.pacificfoods.com
503-692-9666
Fax: 503-692-9610

Sahara Cuisine—Original and organic roasted red pepper hummus made without tahini or oil (other Sahara Cuisine products contain tahini), also black bean dip, lentil dip, and 7-bean dip
PO Box 110866
Cleveland, OH 44111
www.saharacuisineinc.com
216-251-2884

Turtle Mountain—Sweet Nothings fat-free, nondairy fruit-sweetened bars, fudge and mango raspberry
PO Box 21938
Eugene, OR 97402
www.turtlemountain.com
541-338-9400
Fax: 541-338-9401
Consumer inquiries: info@turtlemountain.com

HEALTH FOOD CHAINS

There are many local health food stores, and you may well have good ones nearby. But these three companies have growing networks of stores, and may stock products you are having trouble finding elsewhere. They also carry their own brand-name products that may fit your needs. Trader Joe's, for instance, makes a no-oil pasta sauce, organic spaghetti with mushrooms, and Whole Foods makes its own fat-free pasta sauce and an organic vegan veggie burger that contains no oil. Below is contact information to help you reach their headquarters.

Trader Joe's
800 S. Shamrock Ave.
Monrovia, CA 91016
www.traderjoes.com
626-599-3700

Whole Foods
550 Bowie St.
Austin, TX 78703
www.wholefoodsmarket.com
512-477-4455

Wild Oats Natural Marketplace
3375 Mitchell La.
Boulder, CO 80301
www.wildoats.com
1-800-494-9453

Appendix III

Publications on Heart Disease by the Author

"Beyond Surgery," Presidential Address presented at the Twelfth Annual Meeting of the American Association of Endocrine Surgeons, San Jose, CA, April 14–16, 1991. *Surgery,* December 1991; 110(6):923–27.

with S. G. Ellis, S. V. Medendorp, and T. D. Crowe. "A Strategy to Arrest and Reverse Coronary Artery Disease: A Five-Year Longitudinal Study of a Single Physician's Practice." *The Journal of Family Practice,* December 1995; 41(6):560–68.

(as guest editor) "A Symposium: Summit on Cholesterol and Coronary Disease. 2nd National Conference on Lipids in the Elimination and Prevention of Coronary Disease." Supplement based on a symposium held on September 4–5, 1997, in Lake Buena Vista, FL. *The American Journal of Cardiology,* November 26, 1998; 82(10B):1T–94T.

"Foreword: Changing the Treatment Paradigm for Coronary Artery Disease." *The American Journal of Cardiology,* November 26, 1998; 82(10B):1T–4T.

"Introduction: More Than Coronary Artery Disease." *The American Journal of Cardiology,* November 26, 1998; 82(10B):5T–9T.

"Updating a Twelve-Year Experience with Arrest and Reversal Therapy for Coronary Heart Disease." *The American Journal of Cardiology,* August 1, 1999; 84:339–341.

"In Cholesterol Lowering, Moderation Kills." *Cleveland Clinic Journal of Medicine,* August 2000; 67(8):560–564.

"Resolving the Coronary Artery Disease Epidemic Through Plant-Based Nutrition." *Preventive Cardiology,* 2001; 4:171–177.

Index

Page numbers in italics indicate figures.